Eating Disorders: Prevalence and Treatment

EATING DISORDERS:

Prevalence and Treatment

Edited by SW Touyz and PJV Beumont

WILLIAMS & WILKINS · ADIS PTY LIMITED
Sydney · Baltimore · London

Eating Disorders: Prevalence and Treatment

National Library of Australia
Cataloguing-in-publication data

Eating disorders.

Includes index.
ISBN 0.86433 018 9

1. Anorexia nervosa – Addresses, essays, lectures.
2. Bulimarexia – Addresses, essays, lectures. 3.
Obesity – Addresses, essays, lectures. 4. Appetite
disorders – Addresses, essays, lectures. I. Touyz,
Stephen W. II. Beumont, Pierre J.V.

616.85'2

Printed in Australia by Star Printery Pty. Limited, Erskineville N.S.W.

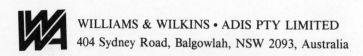

WILLIAMS & WILKINS • ADIS PTY LIMITED
404 Sydney Road, Balgowlah, NSW 2093, Australia

Preface.

Eating disorders constitute a major area of psychosomatic medicine and their prevalence in Western countries is a source of general concern. The treatment of eating disorders remains a challenge to clinicians.

This book is the result of a symposium on eating disorders held at the University of Sydney. Many of the contributors are acknowledged experts of international repute. As well as providing an up-to-date review of recent developments in these disorders the book gives practical advice on the management of patients with anorexia nervosa, bulimia and obesity.

It will be of equal interest to general practitioners, clinical psychologists, dieticians, medical students, school counsellors, psychiatrists and nurses.

Stephen Touyz
Peter Beumont
Sydney
April 1985

CONTRIBUTORS

Suzanne F. Abraham,
Senior Lecturer, Department of Obstetrics and Gynaecology, University of Sydney

Peter J.V. Beumont,
Professor of Psychiatry, University of Sydney

Ian D. Caterson,
Staff Specialist in Endocrinology, Royal Prince Alfred Hospital, Sydney

John K. Collins,
Associate Professor of Psychology, Macquarie University

Robert Gertler,
Senior Visiting Psychiatrist, Royal Prince Alfred Hospital

Anne Hall,
Associate Professor, Department of Psychological Medicine, Wellington Clinical School, University of Otago

Gail F. Huon,
School of Psychology, University of New South Wales

David J. Ivison,
Senior Lecturer, Department of Clinical Psychology, University of Sydney

Ross S. Kalucy,
Professor of Psychiatry, Flinders Medical Centre, Bedford Park, South Australia

Philip Ley,
Professor of Clinical Psychology, University of Sydney

Deborah McClure,
Registrar, Royal Prince Alfred Hospital

Catherine Mason,
    Norman Haire Fellow, Department of Obstetrics and Gynaecology,
    University of Sydney

Michael Mira,
    NHMRC Fellow, Department of Obstetrics and Gynaecology, University
    of Sydney

Tim Sowerbutts,
    Sample Survey Centre, University of Sydney

Stephen W. Touyz,
    Senior Clinical Psychologist, Royal Prince Alfred Hospital and Clinical
    Lecturer in Psychiatry, University of Sydney

A. Stewart Truswell,
    Boden Professor of Human Nutrition, University of Sydney

Hazel Williams,
    Consultant Dietitian, Lynton Private Hospital

Acknowledgements

Chapter IV

The follow-up study was supported by a grant from the Medical Research Council of New Zealand.

The author is particularly grateful to Dr Enid Slim, Psychiatrist, Hutt Regional Community Health Services (INK) whose interviewing skills made the study possible.

Chapter VI

The assistance of Theresa Thomas in the collection of data is gratefully acknowledged. Funds for the project were made available under a University of Sydney Research Grant to the second author.

Chapter XI

I would like to express my appreciation to my colleagues, Mr Jim Jupp, Dr Marita McCabe, Dr Jeanna Sutton, Associate Professor Wendy-Louise Walker and Mrs Jeanette Krass, who formed part of the therapeutic team and to the postgraduate students who also collected and analysed some of the data. The research was supported by ARGS Grant No. A28115063.

Chapter XII

I gratefully acknowledge the work reported here which was carried out by members of the Adelaide Obesity Group, whose members include Dr P.E. Harding, Dr B.H. Higgins and Dr A.N. Goss. Some aspects arise from studies supported by an MRC Grant (No. G972/797/C) and NHMRC Grant (77/2116). I would also like to thank Mrs Gayle Nunn for her support and assistance in coordinating the projects.

Table of Contents

Chapter I

The Syndrome of Anorexia Nervosa

Anorexia nervosa is a condition of excessive self-induced weight loss usually found in adolescent girls and young women, and less commonly seen in pre-pubertal children, males and middle-aged persons. It is a complex illness and many factors contribute to its occurrence in the individual patient. Important among these are the pressures that exist in our society concerning eating, abstention and gratification, to which some people react in a maladaptive way.[1] Anorexia nervosa presents a characteristically dynamic and progressive clinical picture. The illness is often associated with pre-existing obsessionality, depression and low self-esteem, and it has major social effects (invalidism, regression and isolation) and serious physical consequences (severe malnutrition, disordered body chemistry and endocrine dysfunction). Successful treatment depends on recognition of the way these various factors interact.

The condition has become much more common over recent decades and it is no longer a rare illness. In developed Western countries as many as 1 in every 100 girls in their late teens and early twenties are probably affected. Because patients usually minimize their symptoms in order to avoid treatment, their medical attendants may be unaware of the severity of the disturbance or the distress occasioned to the sufferer and her family by what is euphemistically described as dieting.

Characteristics of the Disorder

A central feature of the illness is the patient's preoccupation with her body. This is usually expressed as a concern about weight, but closer enquiry shows that body shape and body tone are at least as important. She dreads being fat or flabby. Some patients have a truely distorted body image, manifested by a persistent overestimation of their size. Although this phenomenon is not pathognomonic of anorexia nervosa (it also occurs in other young women) its recognition is important. Unless the body image misperception is corrected, a real or lasting cure is unlikely.[2]

The illness inevitably involves a number of disturbances of behaviour, all directed at making the patient thin.[3] They include the choice of low-energy foods, increasing abstinence and eventual food refusal; strenuous exercising and restless overactivity; and the use of more bizarre means of weight reduction such as self-induced vomiting, purgation and the abuse of diuretics, laxatives and appetite suppressants.[4] There is great variation between patients in the prominence accorded to each of these behavioural deviations.

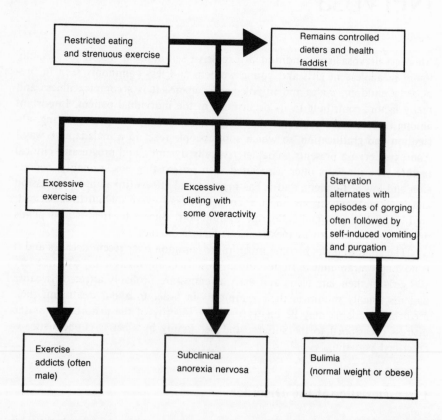

Fig. 1.1 A proposed catagorization of anorexia nervosa and related disorders (based upon an analysis of the behavioural disturbance).

Diagnosis

The major issue of diagnosis is not to differentiate anorexia nervosa from other physical or psychiatric illnesses that cause weight loss, but rather to distinguish it from normal and perhaps even healthy patterns of living such as persistent dietary restraint and committed but reasonable exercising. Patients differ from normal subjects not so much in the types of behaviour they display, but in their addiction to those behaviours – the relentless way in which they pursue them and their inability to desist.

Conditions related to anorexia are shown in figure 1.1. The patient may progress from one category to another. 'Obligatory exercising' or exercise addiction[5] is becoming increasingly common in Australia, and not infrequently progresses to true anorexia nervosa. Similarly, long-continued and excessively restrained eating, the 'dieting' type of anorexia nervosa, may eventually lead to episodes of reactive hyperphagia. Once the patient realizes she can still control her weight by vomiting after each binge, the syndrome of bulimia is established.[6]

Anorexia nervosa is sometimes coincidental with other psychiatric illnesses (schizophrenia, obsessional neurosis) or physical conditions (diabetes mellitus), but in the vast majority of cases it is the primary disorder and the associated physical and psychiatric symptoms are secondary to it. However, these secondary symptoms may demand so much attention that the diagnosis is missed.[7] This mistake will be avoided if the clinician keeps in mind the central importance of the patient's relentless pursuit of thinness. He should also realize that the illness consists primarily of a behavioural disturbance, and that severe emaciation is often only a late manifestation.

Weight Loss

The nutritional disturbance is different to that of protein – calorie malnutrition or starvation. Anorexia nervosa patients usually choose a diet which is very low in energy-dense foods, but relatively high in proteins.[8] Weight loss at first is almost entirely due to loss of adipose tissue and only when fat reserves are exhausted is a significant amount of protein tissue broken down. In an average woman 20% to 30% of the total body mass consists of fat.[9] Therefore, lipid catabolism predominates until the person has reduced to a weight of about 80% of standard or average weight for height. Increased exercise, so characteristic of anorexia nervosa, not only enhances the weight loss but further ensures that it is fat rather than protein that is catabolized.

Most people who diet stop before their energy reserves are seriously depleted. They may suffer minor physiological disturbances such as menstrual disorder and anovulation, euphemistically called hypothalamic amenorrhoea, but they are not ill and are best categorized as having subclinical anorexia nervosa. The point at which fat catabolism no longer suffices fo supply energy needs corresponds closely to the criterion of a weight loss of 20% to 25% required by most classificatory systems for the diagnosis of anorexia nervosa.[10-12]

When the patient's weight falls below that level about three-quarters of available fat tissue has been used up. Protein catabolism now increases markedly, but the decrease in total body mass implies a decreased energy demand, so that an unstable balance is sometimes maintained at a weight of about 65% of standard. In other cases energy intake is further reduced as eating behaviour deteriorates, physiological functioning becomes severely disrupted and weight continues to fall to levels as low as 40% of standard or average weight.

The Physical Disorder

Adipose tissue has a low water content. Consequently there is little disturbance to electrolyte balance during the early phase of the illness. However, when protein catabolism accelerates water is lost, particularly from the intracellular compartment, leading to a fall in total body potassium. Hypokalaemia is rapidly worsened in patients who abuse diuretics or induce vomiting, and a hypochloraemic alkalosis frequently ensues. In some patients the eating disturbance eventually leads to fluid refusal and dehydration, while others try to suppress their hunger by drinking too much fluid and develop water intoxication. Hypernatraema is more common than hyponatraemia.

In mild cases, fat tissue has been lost but muscle bulk is maintained. Despite their illness, many patients are restless and apparently unable to relax. Cold intolerance and acrocyanosis are usual. The skin is dry and scaley (follicular keratitis) and there is an overgrowth of fine downy hair on the face and extensor surfaces (lanugo). Those who have exercised excessively may have sustained stress fractures or dislocations, while the repeated induction of vomiting causes severe dental decay.

In more serious instances emaciation is extreme and the patient is wasted. She is dehydrated and smells acetotic. The mucous membranes are pale and the patient bruises easily. She has a pronounced bradycardia and hypothermia. Peripheral oedema is usually present and may be severe. Occasionally cardiac arrhythmias occur due to hypokalaemia.

Special investigations reveal a moderate normochromic anaemia with reversible bone marrow hypoplasia.[13] The electrolyte disorder has already been discussed. Fatty degeneration of the liver leads to disturbed hepatic function with elevated SGOT, LDH and alkaline phosphatase levels. Cholesterol levels are often raised, reflecting a rise in low-density lipoprotein. Serum albumin may be reduced. Some patients develop pancreatitis during refeeding and serum amylase levels become raised.[14] Acute gastric dilatation and intussusception are other rare complications of treatment.[15]

Endocrine Disturbance

Undernutrition causes a disorder of endocrine function. Failure to recognize this fact has resulted in a great number of patients with anorexia nervosa being unnecessarily investigated for non-existent endocrine disease.[16] Not only are such investigations wasteful, but they may be harmful. They encourage the patient to deny that her problems are due to her disturbed behaviour, and hence allow her to continue to avoid treatment. Such unfortunate developments may be avoided if the medical attendant pays careful attention to the characteristic pattern of endocrine dysfunction that the patient presents.

Amenorrhoea is invariable in anorexia nervosa. It occurs early and often persists long after weight has been restored. It is associated with low oestrogen levels and a decreased secretion of pituitary LH,[17] itself due to inadequate stimulation by the releasing hormone LHRH.[18] Other factors are also involved, particularly an altered sensitivity of the hypothalamic feedback mechanism.[19] The disorder leads to anovular infertility which helps to protect the woman from becoming pregnant while undernourished. The practice of inducing pregnancy by pulsatile LHRH in mild cases of anorexia nervosa with so-called 'hypothalamic amenorrhoea' is questionable in view of the reported association between maternal undernutrition and prematurity.[20]

In male patients, LH and testosterone are depressed and libido is decreased.[21]

Growth hormone[22] and plasma cortisol levels are elevated and the dexamethasone suppression test yields positive results.[23] The raised growth hormone level is necessary to combat hypoglycaemia. These abnormalities are rapidly corrected by refeeding. Patients usually show evidence of mild hypothyroidism with delayed ankle reflexes. While TSH and T4 levels are normal, there is an altered peripheral metabolism of T3 leading to depressed levels of T3 and raised levels of biologically inactive reversed T3.[24] The phenomenon appears to be a compensatory mechanism which serves to minimize energy expenditure. Abnormal GTTs result either from poor absorption or altered insulin response.[25] Both fasting hypoglycaemia and a diabetic curve may be found.

Despite the dietary deficiency and the low oestrogen levels, osteopaenia is relatively uncommon in patients with chronic anorexia. However, a serious consequence of the illness when it occurs in children at around the time of puberty is persistent stunting of growth. There is great variation between patients of similar ages in the extent to which growth is retarded, but it is still unclear why some are more severely affected than others.

Psychiatric Features

In a high proportion of cases the patient's premorbid personality has been characterized by perfectionism and a need to conform. Many have experienced feelings of inability to control their lives, and dieting provides them with their first opportunity to assert their independence. As the illness persists this sense of control is lost and the patient becomes trapped in preoccupations with weight and diet. Underlying obsessionality is exaggerated[26] and spreads to include perfectionistic attitude to school or work and abstention from all enjoyment and relaxation.

The patient is overcome with guilt when she allows herself to enjoy food. Consequently meal times become distressful, she is embarrassed when observed and angry if comments are made about her eating.[27] She deals with food in an obsessional manner, taking an exceedingly long time over meals. Her continued preoccupation is manifested by increasing interest in preparing food for others and in the hoarding of food in caches.

With increasing malnutrition sleep is disturbed, and the patient becomes irritable and depressed.[28] Although she may recognize that she is ill, she is reluctant to admit it. She quarrels with her family about eating, and becomes withdrawn and isolated. Eventually the depression worsens and suicide is a serious risk in chronic cases.

Some patients develop reactive episodes of hyperphagia (bulimia) about which they feel exceedingly guilty.[29] Once patients have learnt to induce vomiting to rid themselves of the unwanted calories, the bulimic episodes serve to reduce tension and hence are difficult to relinquish.

Invalidism

Adolescence is a crucial stage of psychosocial development. Patients with anorexia nervosa are prevented by their illness from accomplishing the developmental tasks of separation from the parental family and establishment of adequate peer relationships. Furthermore, their libido is decreased and sexual development delayed.[30] These factors, particularly when they occur in a person with a rather introverted, rigid and obsessional personality,[26] result in increasing investment in the illness to the exclusion of outside interests. As the illness persists, the patient falls behind her peer group so that socialization becomes progressively more difficult.

The Family

There is often a family history of addictive behaviour (alcohol, tobacco) and of affective disorders.[31]

In a high proportion of cases the patient comes from an affluent background, with professional occupations perhaps being over-represented among parents. However, this middle-class bias is certainly not invariable and anorexia nervosa frequently occurs in working-class families.[32] A group which appears to be particularly at risk is the first-generation offspring of southern European migrants for whom there is considerable dissonance between the expectations of parents and peer group in respect to the role – and figure – of an adolescent girl.

The assessment of family relationships is complicated by 2 factors. First, having a child with anorexia nervosa undoubtedly affects the functioning of the family. Second, as so often is the case with psychiatric illness, parents blame themselves for the daughter's illness. Their guilt is fostered by hearing unsubstantiated theories attributing the illness to faults in parenting. It is worth noting that a recent study failed to find significant premorbid differences between the families of patients with anorexia nervosa and controls.[33]

Parents are worried and bewildered by the patient's behaviour, angry at her obstinate refusal to change and filled with guilt about their perceived role in causing the disturbance. Their consequent ambivalence towards the patient prevents them from being effective in helping her to alter her behaviour, but makes it difficult for them to hand over responsibility for her care to someone else.

As with any other illness, anorexia nervosa can be used by the patient for secondary gain. Because of the illness, the patient attains a privileged position amongst her siblings. In older patients who may be married, the illness is associated with decreased sexual activity and a dependent relationship with the spouse. Sometimes the husband or other relatives place pressure on the patient to conceive, in the hope that this will help her recover. On close enquiry, most patients admit that they are frightened of assuming the responsibilities of motherhood, and that the persistence of their illness is at least partially motivated by their desire to avoid sexual contact and pregnancy. Those who do have children or adopt them often have difficulties in child rearing, particularly in regard to feeding, and it is probably unwise to encourage a patient with anorexia nervosa to adopt a motherhood role before she has successfully overcome her own eating difficulties.

Treatment

The treatment of patients with anorexia nervosa is difficult and controversial. Insulin therapy and psychosurgery are now known to be unwarranted. Various drug regimes have been suggested, such as phenothiazines, the antiserotinergic drug cyproheptadine and the dopamine precursor levodopa, but probably none confers significant benefit.[34,35] Antidepressant medication is sometimes indicated, but only if clinical evidence of concomitant depression is present. While psychotherapy is an important component of treatment, it is of limited value if used on its own, and best if it is of a supportive rather than of an interpretative kind. Active proponents of psychoanalysis admit that their therapy is usually ineffective unless combined with other forms of management,[36] while family therapy as a sole approach has proved disappointing.[37]

There is now substantial agreement that attention to refeeding and the restoration of a normal body weight is mandatory if treatment is to be successful, and refeeding is the key aspect of intervention.[3] The optimal way to bring about weight gain is through admission to a hospital unit where patients are continuously encouraged to eat a high-energy, balanced diet of approximately 14,650 kilojoules per day, under the supervision of skilled nursing staff and using behavioural techniques preferably to reward weight gain rather than eating *per se.*[38] Patients benefit from reassurance about nutritional matters, and the presence of a trained dietician in the therapeutic team is a considerable asset. Forced feeding should never be used.

Refeeding is only the first component of treatment. A major difficulty is the patient's reluctance to return to a normal body weight and shape. Until this attitude is altered, the therapist is likely to be confronted with non-compliance. Therefore, changing the patients abnormal appreciation of her situation must be seen as a crucial task, to be tackled early in treatment. The clinician's skill as a psychotherapist, the persuasive powers of the nursing staff and constant reinforcement provided by healthy peer pressure must all be directed to this aim. If it is not accomplished, no real and lasting cure will be achieved.

After refeeding, most patients require long-term supportive psychotherapy if they are eventually to revert to a normal pattern of behaviour and deal satisfactorily with the developmental problems of adolescence, such as adopting an adult role vis-a-vis their parents, establishing peer relationships and preparing themselves for their future role in society.

Prognosis

Prognosis remains unsatisfactory. Although most experienced therapists, employing the methods above, are able to bring about weight restoration in the short term in approximately 90% of their patients, the relapse rate is high, quoted figures ranging from 35% to 88%.[39] Consequently, the illness usually runs a prolonged course even in the 75% of patients in whom the long-term outcome is eventually favourable.[40] Moreover, a sizeable proportion of patients remain chronic, go on to the related bulimia nervosa, develop other psychiatric illnesses, or die prematurely.

References

1. Garner, D.H. and Garfinkel, P.E.: Sociocultural factors in anorexia nervosa. *Lancet* 2: 674 (1978).
2. Bruch, H.: Perceptual and conceptual disturbances in anorexia nervosa. *Psychological Medicine* 24: 187-94 (1962).
3. Russell, G.F.M.: The present status of anorexia nervosa (editorial) *Psychological Medicine* 7: 363-7 (1977).
4. Beumont, P.J.V., George, G.C. and Smart, D.E.: 'Dieters' and 'vomiters' and 'purgers' in anorexia nervosa. *Psychological Medicine* 6: 617-22 (1976).
5. Yates, A., Leehey, K. and Shisslak, C.M.: Running – An analogue of anorexia? *New England Journal of Medicine* 308(5): 251-5 (1983).
6. Abraham, S.F. and Beumont, P.J.V.: How patients describe bulimia or binge eating. *Psychological Medicine* 12: 625-35 (1982).
7. Beumont, P.J.V.: The endocrinology of anorexia nervosa. *Medical Journal of Australia* 1: 611-13.
8. Beumont, P.J.V., Chambers, T.L., Abrahams, S.F. and Rouse, L.: The diet composition and nutritional knowledge of patients with anorexia nervosa. *Journal of Human Nutrition* 35: 265-731 (1981).
9. Davidson, S., Passmore, R., Brock, J.F. and Truswell, A.S.: *Human Nutrition and Dietetics* 6th ed. p.13 (Churchill Livingstone, Edinburgh 1975).
10. American Psychiatric Association: *Diagnostic and Statistical Manual of Mental Disorders,* 3rd Edn (Washington, 1980).
11. Feighner, J.P., Robins, E., Guze, S.B., Woodruff, R.A. Jr., Winokur, G. and Munoz, R.: Diagnostic criteria for use in psychiatric research. *Archives of General Psychiatry* 26: 57-63 (1972).
12. Russell, G.F.M.: Anorexia nervosa: its identity as an illness and its treatment; in Prive (Ed.) *Modern Trends in Psychological Medicine,* pp.131-64 (Butterworths, London 1970).
13. Mant, M.J. and Faragher, B.S.: The haematology of anorexia nervosa. *British Journal of Haematology* 23: 737-49 (1972).
14. Schoettle, U.C.: Pancreatitis: A complication, a concomitant or a cause of an anorexia nervosa-like syndrome. *Journal of the American Academy of Child Psychiatry* 18: 384-90 (1979).
15. Scobie, B.A.: Acute gastric dilatation and duodenal ileus in anorexia nervosa. *Medical Journal of Australia* 2: 932-4 (1973).
16. Beumont, P.J.V.: Anorexia nervosa: a review. *South African Medical Journal* 44: 911-15 (1970).
17. Beumont, P.J.V., George, G.C.W., Pimstone, B.L. and Vinik, A.I.: The pituitary response to hypothalamic releasing hormones in patients with anorexia nervosa. *Journal of Clinical Endocrinology and Metabolism* 43: 487-96 (1976).
18. Yoshimoto, Y., Moridera, K. and Imura, H.: Restoration of normal pituitary gonadotrophin reserve by administration of luteinizing hormone releasing in patients with hypogonadotrophis hypogonadism. *New England Journal of Medicine* 292: 242-5 (1975).
19. Wakeling, A., de Souza, V.F.A., Gore, M.B.R., Sabur, M., Kingstone, D. and Boss, A.M.B.: Amenorrhoea, body weight and serum hormone concentrations, with particular reference to prolactin and thyroid hormones in anorexia nervosa. *Psychological Medicine* 9: 265-72 (1979).
20. Lind, T.: Would more calories per day keep low birthweight at bay? In: Nutrition: The Changing Scene. *Lancet* 501-2.
21. Beumont, P.J.V., Beardwood, C.J. and Russell, G.F.M.: The occurrence of the syndrome of anorexia nervosa in males. *Psychological Medicine* 2: 216-31 (1971).

22. Vigersky, A. and Loriaux, L.D.: Anorexia nervosa as a model of hypothalamic dysfunction. In: R.A. Vigersky (Ed.) *Anorexia Nervosa* pp.109-22 (Raven Press, New York 1977).

23. Doerr, P., Fichter, M., Pirke, K.M. and Lund, T.: Relationship between weight gain and hypothalamic pituitary adrenal function in patients with anorexia nervosa. *Journal of Steroid Biochemistry* 13: 529-37 (1980).

24. Leslie, R.D.G., Isaacs, A.J., Gomez, J., Raggatt, P.R. and Bayliss, R.: Hypothalamo-pituitary-thyroid function in anorexia nervosa: Influence of weight gain. *British Medical Journal* 2: 526-8 (1978).

25. Wachslicht-Rodbard, H., Gross, H.A., Rodbard, D., Ebert, M.A. and Roth, J.: Increased insulin binding to erythrocytes in anorexia nervosa. Restoration to normal with refeeding. *New England Journal of Medicine* 300: 882-7 (1979).

26. Smart, D.E., Beumont, P.J.V. and George, G.C.W.: Some personality characteristics of patients with anorexia nervosa. *British Journal of Psychiatry* 128: 57-60 (1976).

27. Russell, G.F.M. and Gillies, C.: Investigation and care of patients in a psychiatric metabolic ward. *Nursing Times* 60: 852-4.

28. Crisp, A.H.: Sleep, activity and mood. *British Journal of Psychiatry* 137: 1-7 (1980).

29. Russell, G.F.M.: Bulimia nervosa, an ominous variant of anorexia nervosa. *Psychological Medicine* 9: 429-48 (1979).

30. Beumont, P.J.V., Abraham, S.F., and Simson, K.G.: Sexual experiences and attitudes in girls and women with anorexia nervosa. *Psychological Medicine* 11: 131-40 (1981).

31. Winokur, A., March, V. and Mendels, J.: Primary affective disorder in relatives of patients with anorexia nervosa. *American Journal of Psychiatry* 137: 695-8 (1980).

32. Beumont, P.J.V., Abraham, S.F., Argall, W.J., George, G.C.W. and Glaun, D.E.: The onset of anorexia nervosa. *Australian and New Zealand Journal of Psychiatry* 12: 145-9 (1979).

33. Hall, A., Leibeich, J. and Walkey, F.H.: The development of a food, fitness and looks questionnaire and its use in a study of 'weight pathology' in 204 nonpatient families; in Darby, Garfinkel, Garner and Coscina (Eds). *Anorexia nervosa: Recent Developments in Research* (Alan R. Liss, New York 1983).

34. Dally, P. amd Sargant, W.: A new treatment of anorexia nervosa. *British Medical Journal* 1: 1770-3 (1960).

35. Vigersky, R.A. and Loriaux, D.L.: The effect of cyproheptadine in anorexia nervosa: a double blind trial; in Vigersky (Ed.) *Anorexia nervosa* pp. 349-356 (Raven Press, New York 1977).

36. Bruch, H.: *Eating Disorders,* (Routledge and Kegan Paul, London 1974).

37. Minuchin, S., Rosman, B.L. and Baker, L.: *Psychosomatic Families. Anorexia Nervosa in Context* (Harvard University Press, Cambridge-Massachusetts-London 1978).

38. Touyz, S.W., Gilandas, A.J. and Beumont, P.J.V.: Treating an eating disorder with behavioural techniques; in Tiller and Martin (Eds) *Behavioural Medicine* (Geigy, Sydney 1981).

39. Hsu, L.K.G., Crisp, A.H. and Harding, B.: Outcome of anorexia nervosa. *Lancet* 1: 61-5 (1979).

40. Touyz, S.W. and Beumont, P.J.V.: Anorexia nervosa. A follow-up study *Medical Journal of Australia* 141(4): 219-22 (1984).

41. Crisp, A.H., Palmer, R.L. and Kalucy, R.S.: How common is anorexia nervosa? A prevalence study. *British Journal of Psychiatry* 128: 549-54 (1976).

Chapter II

A Comprehensive, Multidisciplinary Approach for the Management of Patients with Anorexia Nervosa

Anorexia nervosa is a syndrome of self-induced weight loss which usually occurs in adolescent girls and young women. Associated with obsessionality, depression, and low self-esteem, it is characterized by the excessive use of behaviours directed at bringing about weight loss. It has important social implications and often results in regression, invalidism and isolation. Physical manifestations of the disorder include malnutrition, disturbed body chemistry and endocrine dysfunction.[1] Because of the complex interaction of psychological factors in the geneses of the varied symptomatology, it has been called a paradigm of psychosomatic disorders.[2] It was recognized as a syndrome more than a hundred years ago by William Gull,[3] a physician at Guys Hospital who was mainly concerned with the physical manifestations of the disease. It was also described independently by Charles Laseque,[4] a psychiatrist at the Pitie in Paris, who was intrigued by its rich phenomenology and entitled his paper 'De l'anorexie hysterique'. Both authors attributed the onset of anorexia nervosa to psychological factors.

Over the last two decades there has been an increased concern amongst women in contemporary society to maintain slim figures.[5,6] This has been associated with an increase in the incidence of anorexia nervosa.[7,8]

A recent report by Willi and Grossmann, who conducted a retrospective study of the incidence of anorexia nervosa in Zurich, revealed that the incidence of anorexia nervosa increased significantly from 0.38/100 000 for 1956-58 to 0.55/100 000 for 1963-65 to 1.12/100 000 for 1973-75.[9]

Crisp *et al.* reported that 1 out of every 100 school girls over the age of 16 years attending private schools in London is probably affected.[10] The increased occurrence of anorexia nervosa has been accompanied by a greater awareness of the disorder by medical practitioners, clinical psychologists and school counsellors and there is now a tendency to make the diagnosis earlier – before the patient has become severely emaciated.[1]

Despite the increased prevalence of anorexia nervosa, its treatment remains difficult and controversial. Numerous and varied techniques have been advocated. These include insight-oriented psychotherapy,[11] medication,[12] tube feeding,[13] electroconvulsive therapy[14] and even psychosurgery.[15] While behavioural techniques appear to be the most effective means of restoring a normal body weight,[16,17] the relapse rate following treatment remains an area of much concern.[18]

Behaviour Therapy in Anorexia Nervosa

Bachrach *et al.* introduced the concept of using operant techniques in the management of patients admitted to hospital with anorexia nervosa.[19] They treated a 37-year-old woman using social reinforcement (e.g. conversation, attention and praise), which was made contingent upon her eating her meals. In order to maximize weight gain, they placed her in a single room without the usual entertainments such as television and books. Visits from both staff and relatives were restricted. She initially gained weight on this regime, but her weight gain levelled off after she had put on 7.2kg. To encourage further weight gain, they made rewards contingent upon weight gain rather than eating behaviour. Unfortunately the patient was discharged from hospital shortly thereafter, and it is not known whether any further weight gain occurred.

Leitenberg *et al.* replicated the work of Bachrach and his colleagues and they reported that conversation and attention during meals was not successful in producing weight gain.[20] However, when they rewarded weight gain directly, a steady increase in both caloric intake and weight gain was observed. These studies stimulated a great deal of interest in the application of behaviour modification, especially in relationship to weight gain.

Agras and Werne reviewed the literature regarding the application of behavioural technology.[17] They concluded that behavioural techniques resulted in a more consistent weight gain, favourable outcome and less use of coercive methods (e.g. tube feeding and intravenous therapy) than non-behavioural methods of treatment. They suggested that the less frequent use of tube feeding and/or intravenous therapy was associated with lower mortality rates and strongly advocated the use of behaviour therapy in the management of the hospitalized patient with anorexia nervosa.

Bruch, on the other hand, has expressed great concern regarding the use of behaviour modification in anorexia nervosa.[21, 22] In a paper entitled 'Perils of Behaviour Modification in Anorexia Nervosa', she strongly criticized behaviour therapists for their naive assumption that the restoration of a normal body weight (the most prominent symptom) was sufficient treatment. It was her impression that most behaviourally oriented programmes failed to take into account the major deficits in the personality development of these patients, namely low self-esteem, self-doubt, lack of autonomy and an inability to lead a self-directed life. She also indicated that behavioural programmes had an adverse psychological effect on patients who would gain weight under the 'pressure of persuasion, force or threats' and would literally 'eat their way out' of hospital. Bruch concluded by saying that 'it is generally known that true benefit is derived from such weight gain only if it is part of an integrated treatment programme with correction of the underlying individual and family problems'.[22]

With these criticisms in mind, we recently evaluated a behavioural programme which allowed patients to maintain a greater degree of control over their refeeding process.[23] The results were contrasted with the more traditional approach which requires the patient to be confined to bed and have all her possessions removed. An individualized schedule of reinforcers was then drawn up.[24] Sixty-five patients with anorexia nervosa consecutively admitted to an eating disorder clinic, participated in the study. They were divided into 2 cohorts. The first 31 were treated using a strict bed-rest programme with an individualized schedule of reinforcers for each 0.5kg gained. The next 34 patients were treated using a lenient, flexible behavioural programme which will be described in detail under the heading Weight Restoration Programme. Our most important observation was that the mean daily weight gain did not differ significantly between the 2 treatment programmes (0.21 vs 0.20kg/day). The mean daily weight gain on both programmes also compared favourably with the best figures reported by other authors using behavioural techniques. There were practical advantages to using the lenient programme. It was seen as more acceptable by most of our patients, and there was a general consensus among staff members that patients on the lenient programme were better motivated towards treatment and required less nursing care. It was therefore more economical and it provided less opportunity for patients to manipulate individual staff members in connection with their treatment. As a result, the staff were able to use their time more constructively in both group therapy and supportive psychotherapy with the patients. This was very much in keeping with our overall aim of providing a comprehensive integrated approach to treatment.[25]

Our pragmatic multidisciplinary treatment approach has many factors in common with the one described by Anderson *et al.*, with the notable exception being our behavioural rather than psychodynamic emphasis.[26] Anderson *et al.* described their approach in the following manner:

'The assumption is that no single aetiological factor predominates, but, rather, several factors exist which, when combined, give rise to the condition. A multi-factorial orientation underlies this treatment approach. The treatment focus, therefore, is to integrate biological, psychological and family treatment and to modify treatment as experience dictates for individual patients.'

Our overall programme, like those of Garfinkel and Garner[27] and Anderson *et al.*,[26] consists of a series of integrated treatment approaches based on our belief that a number of factors are involved in the causation and persistence of anorexia nervosa. Inportant aspects of the programme are:

1. Regulated weight gain occurs in a warm, supportive environment;
2. Informational feedback and dietary counselling are given on a regular basis;
3. A moderate but graduated level of activity is allowed;
4. Emphasis is given to our view that weight gain is essential but is only part of the overall treatment programme;
5. Occupational therapy, social skills and assertiveness training groups are utilized;
6. Supportive psychotherapy is given on an individual basis;
7. All families are assessed and several taken into family therapy;
8. Ward outings including visits to restaurants are organized by nursing staff on a regular basis;
9. Patients usually return to school or work for a week or two before discharge from the unit.

Assessment for Admission

A detailed personal, social, medical and psychiatric history is taken as well as a comprehensive assessment of diet, eating behaviour and physical activity. In order that full blood count, liver function tests and electrolyte levels can be determined, 10ml blood is taken. Once this information has been obtained, a decision is made about admission to hospital. The following factors are taken into account when making such a decision: the distance the individual has to travel to attend appointments; the degree of emaciation; presence of medical complications; failure to show improvement during previous outpatient therapy and the patient's expressed inability to control either self-induced vomiting or bulimia. If the patient is not too emaciated and is motivated to change maladaptive behaviour patterns, then outpatient treatment would be considered. Such treatment usually consists of supportive psychotherapy which is carried out by a psychiatrist and/or a clinical psychologist, nutritional counselling by a dietitian (chapter 3) and exploration of family or marital problems by a social worker. Individual patients are also offered an opportunity to obtain feedback concerning their present perceived shape (subjective image - figure 2.1) and also their judgement of their ideal shape (optative image - figure 2.2) using a video camera with a distorting lens.[28] Patients also attend a therapeutic group in which they are encouraged to confront and assist one another in overcoming maladaptive attitudes and behaviours, and to discuss interpersonal difficulties in a warm, supportive environment. Individuals are initially seen weekly for supportive psychotherapy and nutritional counselling and this is changed to fortnightly on an individual basis. Approximately 50% of our referrals are treated entirely as outpatients.

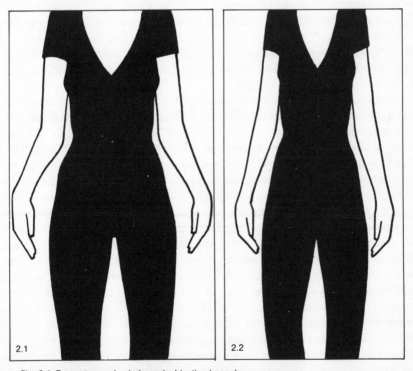

Fig. 2.1 Present perceived shape (subjective image)

Fig. 2.2 Ideal shape (optative image)

Hospital Management

The hospital management of patients with anorexia nervosa can be conveniently divided into stages, i.e. weight restoration (stage 1) and weight maintenance (stage 2). The effects of starvation need to be overcome if the patient is to benefit meaningfully from the other aspects of the programme such as supportive psychotherapy.

Weight Restoration (Stage 1)

On admission to hospital, the behaviourly orientated ward programme is explained to the individual patient by the nursing sister in charge of the unit. The nursing staff on the unit are responsible for the day to day management of the patients and are well versed with the psychopathology of anorexia nervosa. Russell has stressed the importance of nursing staff in the hospital management of patients with anorexia nervosa: '... The greater burden of responsibility for inpatient treatment should be given to the nurses caring for the patients ... the key to the success of nursing care is the establishment of a relationship of trust between the patient and those nurses who will have the closest contact with her.'[29] It is therefore of the utmost importance that the senior nursing staff members make a commitment to work on the unit on a regular basis and that there is not a frequent turnover of staff.

Patients usually spend the first week restricted to the unit, but those individuals who are severely emaciated are restricted to bed rest. Individuals must gain a minimum of 1.5kg per week if they are to avoid bed rest for a further week. When individuals fail to gain the required weight, they realize that they will have to spend the following week restricted to bed rest. Once on bed rest, they keep all their possessions such as books, radio or television, but are not permitted visits from family or friends. The other patients in the unit are allowed to visit. Whilst restricted to bed rest, the patients continue to attend therapeutic groups and continue to eat their meals in the dining room. This approach differs significantly from that of Crisp, who advocates total bed rest for 6 to 8 weeks until the patient reaches the set target weight. [30,31] Individual psychotherapy would continue throughout this time. Garfinkel and Garner initially prefer to keep their patients restricted to bed rest and allow them up as their weight increased.[27] They stress that the amount of time for which each individual is allowed up is dependent upon the patient and the degree of emaciation, but on average allow 1 hour for each kilogram gained. It has been our experience that most patients gain weight whilst on the unit without being restricted to bed rest. As stated previously, this provides less opportunity for patients to manipulate staff members and they can spend their time more constructively attending individual, group and occupational therapy. Peer pressure within the therapeutic community contributes significantly to patients attaining their weekly weight gain. Patients are permitted to sit outside in the garden or go for short walks but are unable to do so if they are restricted to bed rest. As a result, patients encourage one another to eat their prescribed meal plan to ensure the required weight gain.

All family members living in the patient's home are asked to meet with the family therapist just before or shortly after admission. At this interview, an assessment of family interactional patterns is made and a decision regarding family therapy is taken at a weekly ward meeting attended by all members of the multidisciplinary team. Not all families need to have regular therapy and a decision is made for each individual family. If family therapy is considered to be desirable, then the team decides which family members should attend and how frequent the sessions need to be. For example, if the parents of the index patient have marked marital difficulties, the family therapist may choose to work with the parents for a number of sessions before including the patient. The objectives of family intervention are similar to those described by Anderson et al.,[26] namely:

1. To enable the family members to understand the illness and the goals of treatment;
2. A readjustment of family interactional patterns where appropriate; and
3. The participation in post-discharge planning and activities, i.e. it is often most beneficial for the patient and her mother to meet with the dietitian to discuss the resumption of normal eating behaviour when the patient returns home.

The dietitian takes a comprehensive nutritional history shortly after admission[32] and sees the patient on a regular basis for nutritional counselling. Not all programmes include a dietitian and Russell assigns the responsibility for nutritional matters to the nursing staff ' . . . the nurse . . .offers to become responsible for her choice of food and its amount saying: "leave these decisions to me, I can promise that the amount of food chosen for you is what you need and I shall make sure that you do not become fat" '.[29] We find it preferable to include a dietitian who is better equipped to deal with all the issues that arise concerning food and weight. Most patients have developed a rigid choice of food and provide long lists of taboo foods which they religiously avoid. The dietitian insists that patients eat a well-balanced, nutritionally adequate diet and encourages individuals to gradually incorporate taboo foods, e.g. red meat, cakes, chocolates, into their meal plan. To facilitate this, the dietitian prescribes a 'spot meal' each week. The individual is only informed of what the meal comprises when they arrive in the dining room. It is important not to condone anorexic eating behaviour (i.e. large plates of salads with low fat yoghurt) and to include energy-dense foods as well. We do not prescribe vitamins and reassure patients that they will obtain sufficient quantities of vitamins by eating a well-balanced diet. It has previously been suggested that patients with anorexia nervosa as a group specifically avoid carbohydrates.[30] However, a careful analysis of their nutritional intake by Chambers *et al.* revealed that they had a relatively low intake of fats which contributed an average of only 36% of their energy intake during the initial stages of weight loss.[33] As dieting and weight loss progressed, the relative proportion of fats in their diets decreased to 27% of energy intake, while that of carbohydrates actually increased from 43% to 55%, despite an over-all reduction in the intake of all nutrients. The relative proportion of protein was high, about 22% of energy intake throughout the dieting period.

The initial caloric intake prescribed for each individual varies as it is dependent upon their intake just prior to admission. Gastric dilatation may occur if refeeding is too rapid in a severely emaciated patient.[27] Most patients are initially prescribed a 4200 to 6300 kilojoule diet and this is gradually increased to approximately 14 650 kilojoules per day. The number of kilojoules per day required to ensure consistent weight gain varies greatly between individual patients. Those individuals who require greater than 14 650 kilojoules per day are encouraged to add a high-energy compound, Polyjoule,® to their meal plan. Because of the possible iatrogenic contribution to the development of bulimia, patients should not be encouraged to consume excessively large quantities of food at meal times. In addition, patients are advised not to eat more than their prescribed diet and are not permitted to hoard food or have relatives bring food into the ward.[34]

Staff members are encouraged to eat meals with the patients to provide a model for normal healthy attitudes towards food and appropriate eating behaviour. From time to time, videotapes are made of the patients eating their meals and these are played back to them in a group setting. Abnormal eating behaviours are pointed out and ways of improving them are discussed by the group. Agras *et al.* reported that 'informational feedback is more important in the treatment of anorexia nervosa than positive reinforcement, while serving of large meals is least important'.[35] We deliberately do not prescribe excessively large meals as this encourages abnormal eating patterns, but rather insist that individuals eat all the food on their prescribed diet.

Patients are weighed daily at 7:00 a.m. and are told their daily weight gain or lack thereof. This feedback is extremely important for patients as they are usually most concerned that they will gain weight too rapidly. Patients are required to rest on their beds for 30 minutes following breakfast and for an hour after both lunch and dinner. Patients with a previous history of self-induced vomiting are often tempted to do so after a meal whereas those who have been excessively active (exercising) prior to admission are inclined to pay back the debt (meal consumed) by exercising strenuously. Bed rest can be seen as 'response prevention' in behavioural terms. Patients are told that both vomiting and over-exercising are unacceptable and they are to consult with members of the nursing staff when they get the urge to do so.

The patients' target weights are determined by the consultant, who refers to a chart of desirable body weights[36] and patients are given a desirable range and are encouraged to maintain their weight within this range. Patients are usually given their target weight range once they have started gaining weight. Target weights can also be determined by arbitrarily selecting a weight that is 90% of standard body weight for the individual's age and height,[37] or by means of a matched population weight.[31] The patient should be reassured that she won't be forced or even allowed to become obese. However, care must be taken to avoid being trapped into promises of keeping the patient's weight at an abnormally low level.[38] Garfinkel and Garner suggest that the patient's target weight should be marginally higher than her previously 'tolerable upper limit' in order for her to overcome her irrational concerns about having a larger shape.[27] It is also most important that the patient not have to diet in order to maintain a target weight.

Patients receive regular individual supportive psychotherapy sessions and attend psychotherapy groups, e.g. social skills, assertiveness training and problem solving groups. Patients who complain of anxiety symptoms and tension receive relaxation therapy. Medication is prescribed infrequently.

Psychotherapy should be of a supportive and directive nature rather than of an insight-oriented interpretive kind. Bruch, who reported on 43 patients, initially treated her patients using a psychodynamic approach, but eventually conceded that this type of treatment was conspicuously ineffective in the management of patients with anorexia nervosa.[39]

Patients also receive weekly feedback about their judgement of their body image using a video camera with a distorting lens.[28]

The duration of weight restoration is variable but usually occurs within 6 to 8 weeks. This is followed by the weight maintenance programme.

Weight Maintenance (Stage 2)

The duration of the weight maintenance period is usually 2 to 3 weeks. During this period, the patient reduces her kilojoule intake under the supervision of the dietitian from approximately 14 650 kilojoules per day to a maintenance level of about 7550 to 9200 kilojoules per day.

Once this is achieved, individuals are encouraged to eat out at restaurants with family and friends and to spend evenings and weekends at home. They are permitted to go shopping and are encouraged to buy a new wardrobe of clothes. Once the individual has successfully reduced her kilojoule intake to a maintenance level arrangements are made for her to return to school or work and most individuals would do so for a week to 10 days prior to discharge. Supportive psychotherapy and nutritional counselling continues throughout this period and a family therapy session is also arranged just before or after discharge.

During the weight maintenance period, patients are weighed 2 or 3 times per week to ensure that they are maintaining their weight above the minimum acceptable target weight. They are told that if their weight should drop below their target range, they have to remain restricted to bed rest until they have regained the lost weight.

Those individuals who have had to gain a substantial amount of weight may develop a distended abdomen. This is usually a source of great concern and has an adverse effect upon the individual who is trying to come to terms with a larger figure. In such instances, it is well worthwhile referring the patient to a physiotherapist or to a gymnasium if it is conveniently located, so that specific exercises can be prescribed to tone up abdominal muscles. Those individuals who have lost weight, because of an inability to control the amount of exercise they have, should only do so under strict supervision.[40]

Once the weight maintenance period has been completed, patients are discharged from hospital and continue to attend the unit as outpatients. They should initially be seen on a weekly or fortnightly basis and attend an outpatient group as many patients who have been admitted to hospital with anorexia nervosa relapse within 6 months of leaving hospital.

Summary

The treatment of anorexia nervosa remains difficult and controversial and numerous treatments have been suggested over the years. There is now a general consensus that the restoration of a normal body weight is mandatory if treatment is to be successful.

References

1. Beumont, P.J.V. and Russell, J.: Anorexia nervosa; in Beumont and Burrows (Eds) *Handbook of Psychiatry and Endocrinology* pp. 63-96 (Elsevier Biomedical Press, Amsterdam 1982).
2. Kaufman, R.M. and Heiman, M. (Eds): *Evolution of Psychosomatic Concepts: Anorexia Nervosa: A Paradigm*. International Universities Press, New York 1964).
3. Gull, W.W.: Anorexia nervosa. Trans. Clinical Society (London) 7: 22-8 (1974). Reprinted in Kaufman and Heiman (Eds) *Evolution of Psychosomatic Concepts. Anorexia Nervosa: A Paradigm* (International Universities Press, New York 1964).
4. Laseque, C.: De l'anorexie hysterique. *Arch. Gen du Med.* 385 (1973) reprinted in Kaufman and Heiman (Eds) *Evolution of Psychosomatic Concepts. Anorexia Nervosa: A Paradigm.* (International Universities Press, New York 1964).
5. Garner, D.M. and Garfinkel, P.E.: Sociocultural factors in anorexia nervosa. *Lancet* 2: 674 (1978).
6. Abraham, S.F., Mira, M., Beumont, P.J.V., Sowerbutts, T.D. and Llewellyn-Jones, D.: Eating behaviours among young women. *Medical Journal of Australia.* 24: 225-8 (1983).

7. Kendell, R.E., Hall, D.J., Hailey, A. and Babigan, H.M. The epidemiology of anorexia nervosa. *Psychological Medicine*, 3: 200-3 (1973).
8. Jones, D.J., Fox, M.M., Babigan, H.M. and Hutten, H.E.: Epidemiology of anorexia nervosa in Monroe Country, New York (1960-1976) *Psychosomatic Medicine* 42: 551-8 (1980).
9. Willi, J. and Grossman, S.: Epidemiology of anorexia nervosa in a defined region of Switzerland. *American Journal of Psychiatry* 240 (5): 564-7 (1983).
10. Crisp, A.H. Palmer, R., and Kalucy, R.S.: How common is anorexia nervosa? A prevalence study. *British Journal of Psychiatry* 128: 549-54 (1976).
11. Bruch, H.: *Eating Disorders: Obesity, Anorexia Nervosa and the Person Within*. (Basic Books, New York 1974).
12. Dally, P.J. and Sargent, W.: A new treatment of anorexia nervosa. *British Medical Journal* 1: 1770-3 (1960).
13. Silverman, J.A.: Clinical observations in a successful treatment plan. *Journal of Paediatrics* 84: 68-73 (1974).
14. Laboucarie, J. and Barres, P.: Les aspects cliniques, pathogeniques et therapeutiques de l'anorexie mentale. *L'Evolution Psychiat.* 1: 119-46 (1954).
15. Crisp, A. and Kalucy, R.S.: The effect of leucotomy in intractable adolescent weight phobia (primary anorexia nervosa). *Postgraduate Medical Journal* 49: 833-93 (1973).
16. Touyz, S.W., Gilandas, A.J. and Beumont, P.J.V.: Treating an eating disorder with behavioural techniques; in Tiller and Martin *Geigy Psychiatric Symposium on Behavioural Medicine* 9: 173-7 (1980).
17. Agras, W.S. and Werne, J.: Behaviour therapy in anorexia nervosa: A data-based approach to the question; in Brady and Brodie (Eds) *Controversy in Psychiatry* (WB Saunders Publishing Co. Philadelphia 1978).
18. Hsu, L.K.G.: Outcome of anorexia nervosa. A review of the literature (1954-1978). *Archives of General Psychiatry*, 37: 1041-6 (1980).
19. Bachrach, A.J. Erwin, W.J. and Mohr, J.P.: The control of eating behaviour in an anorexic by operant conditioning techniques; in Ullmann and Krasner (Eds) *Case Studies in Behaviour Modification* (Holt Rinehart and Winston, New York 1965).
20. Leitenberg, H., Agras, W.S. and Thomson, L.E.: A sequential analysis of the effect of selective positive reinforcement in modifying anorexia nervosa. *Behaviour Research and Therapy* 6: 211-18 (1968).
21. Bruch, H.: Perils of behaviour modification in treatment of anorexia nervosa. *Journal of the American Medical Association*, 230(10): 1419-22 (1974).
22. Bruch, H.: Dangers of behaviour modification in treatment of anorexia nervosa; in Brady and Brodie (Eds) *Controversy in Psychiatry* (WB Saunders Co. Philadelphia 1978).
23. Russell, G.F.M.: Anorexia Nervosa: Its identity as an illness and its treatment; in Prior (Ed.) *Modern Trends in Psychological Medicine*, 2. (Butterworths, London 1970).
24. Touyz, S.W., Beumont, P.J.V., Glaun, D., Philips, T. and Cowie, I.: A comparison of lenient and strict operant conditioning programmes in refeeding patients with anorexia nervosa. *British Journal of Psychiatry* 144:512-20 (1984).
25. Touyz, S.W. and Beumont, P.J.V.: The use of multimodal therapy in the treatment of anorexia nervosa. *Australian Clinical Psychologist* 16(1): 23-32 (1984).
26. Anderson, A.E. Hedblom, J.E. and Hubbard, F.A.: A multidisciplinary team treatment for patients with anorexia nervosa and their families. *International Journal of Eating Disorders*, 2(4): 181-92 (1983).
27. Garfinkel, P.E. and Garner, D.M.: *Anorexia Nervosa: A Multidimensional Perspective*. (Brunner/Hazel, New York 1982).
28. Touyz, S.W., Beumont, P.J.V., Collins, J.K., McCabe, M. and Jupp, J.: Body shape perception and its disturbance in anorexia nervosa. *British Journal of Psychiatry* 144: 167-71 (1984).

29. Russell, G.F.M.: General management of anorexia nervosa and difficulties in assessing the efficacy of treatment; in Vigersky (Ed.) *Anorexia Nervosa,* pp.281 (Raven Press, New York 1977).

30. Crisp, A.H.: Clinical and therapeutic aspects of anorexia nervosa - a study of thirty cases. *Journal of Psychosomatic Research* 9: 67-78 (1965).

31. Crisp, A.H.: Premorbid factors in adult disorders of weight, with particular reference to primary anorexia nervosa (weight phobia). A literature review. *Journal of Psychosomatic Research* 14: 1-22 (1970).

32. Beumont, P.J.V., Chambers, T.L., Rouse, L. and Abraham, S.F.: The diet composition and nutritional knowledge of patients with anorexia nervosa. *Journal of Human Nutrition* 35: 265-73 (1981).

33. Chambers, T.L., Beumont, P.J.V. and Abraham, S.F.: The diet histories and nutrient intakes of anorexia nervosa patients. *Food and Nutrition Notes and Reviews.* Australian Commonwealth, Department of Health, 356: 64-65 (1979).

34. Frankenburg, F.R.: Hoarding in anorexia nervosa. *British Journal of Medical Psychology* 57: 57-60 (1984).

35. Agras, W.S., Barlow, D.H., Chapin, H.N., Abel, G.G., Jackson, M., Leitenberg, H. and Burlington, V.: Behaviour modification of anorexia nervosa. *Archives of General Psychiatry* 30:279-86 (1974).

36. Society of Actuaries: *Build and Blood Pressure Study* (Society of Actuaries, Itasca, Illinois 1959).

37. Sorlie, P., Gordon, T. and Kannel, W.B.: Body build and mortality: The Framingham Study. *Journal of the American Medical Association,* 243: 1828-31 (1980).

38. Beumont, P.J.V.: Anorexia nervosa: A review. *South African Medical Journal* 44 (August): 911-15 (1970).

39. Bruch, H.: Anorexia nervosa and its differential diagnosis. *Journal of Nervous and Mental Diseases,* 141: 555-66 (1966).

40. Beumont, P.J.V., Touyz, S.W. and Hook, S.: Excessive exercise in anorexia nervosa. Proceedings of the International Conference on Anorexia Nervosa and Related Disorders, Swansea 1984.

Chapter III

Nutritional Counselling in Anorexia Nervosa

Nutritional counselling has not usually been included in the treatment of anorexia nervosa,[1] which has been seen primarily as a psychiatric disorder. However, patients with anorexia nervosa develop many abnormal eating behaviours and incorrect beliefs about food which need to be corrected if these individuals are to return to a normal, nutritious eating pattern.[2-4]

The nutritional therapist, or dietitian, can make a significant contribution in treating patients with anorexia nervosa. Detailed nutritional and behavioural information can be collected which may be used by all members of the treatment team in their assessment and management of the patient. The dietitian can provide a necessary structure to the refeeding phase of treatment by prescribing and supervising daily meals, and can guide the rehabilitation of the patients back to selection of appropriate meals for weight maintenance. Another important area where nutritional counselling is often required is with the families of patients with anorexia nervosa. The difficulties the individual has experienced concerning food are discussed as well as those that may be anticipated after discharge from hospital. Throughout the treatment period, nutritional education can be of great value to correct the distorted ideas that patients develop about food, and to provide a professional point of view on healthy eating patterns.

We will describe the idea of the dietitian as a nutritional counsellor and educator within a multidisciplinary treatment programme.[5] Development and the therapeutic value of such counselling is critically examined.

Nutritional Assessment

Nutritional information is collected primarily in the form of a diet and weight history, taken verbally from the patients, but checked upon and added to at later stages in their treatment. All dietitians are trained to take such histories and can translate them into levels of nutrient and energy intakes during the development of the eating disorder. Information is also collected about the behaviours used by patients to reduce their energy intake and weight, the development of the patients' beliefs and fears about food, and their level of nutritional knowledge. Examples of some behaviours commonly used by patients with anorexia nervosa to lose weight are:

1. Reduce all food intake;
2. Reduce selectively high energy foods;
3. Try various 'fad' diets;
4. Eat predominantly high bulk, low energy foods;
5. Miss meals (usually lunch for school girls);
6. Self-induced vomiting;
7. Starvation (sometimes alternating with periods of gorging and vomiting);
8. Use commerical 'dietary' foods such as artificial sweeteners, skimmed milk cheese and yoghurt;
9. Pick continuously in place of meals;
10. Chew food and spit it out;
11. Excessive activity.

The dietitian uses the diet history to pinpoint specific areas for nutritional counselling and as a guide for the size of diet required to initiate weight gain. A nutritional base state at admission is also provided by the diet history, which can be useful for comparing similar parameters at discharge and follow-up. Throughout the admission period the dietitian observes the patient eating, to obtain information about their food choices and eating behaviour at the table. This often reveals abnormal eating behaviours that the patient may not have admitted to, or even recognized as detrimental to their recovery. Such observed behaviours are:

1. Eating slowly;
2. Cutting food into very small mouthfuls;
3. Using small utensils;
4. Hiding food at the table;
5. Elaborate food preparation procedures, often handling food excessively;
6. Precise measurement of food at every meal;
7. Leaving the table frequently during a meal;
8. Keeping to a rigid eating pattern of very few foods;
9. Denying hunger, tiredness and other symptoms of starvation;
10. Avoiding social occasions where eating may be involved;

11. Difficulty in making choices about what to eat;
12. Smoking cigarettes;
13. Cooking for others, sometimes controlling the family kitchen and commanding how the family eats.

The dietitian would discuss these behaviours with individual patients and suggest more appropriate, socially acceptable alternatives. At some stage of treatment, the patient's parents or spouse, where appropriate, are interviewed by the dietitian to help verify and complete the diet history.

The Refeeding Programme

Weight gain is usually achieved in treatment programmes for patients with anorexia nervosa,[6] but weight gain alone may not alter the patient's abnormal eating behaviours or their attitudes to eating and food.[7] This aspect of treatment is often ignored with the assumption that it will correct itself as weight is normalized.[8] In our experience this is not always so. If left to themselves, patients with anorexia nervosa may increase their total energy input but will invariably keep their food choice limited to the few 'safe' foods they were eating before treatment. Similarly, their attitudes and beliefs about food will remain little changes unless aired, discussed and corrected by a professional with a specialized training in nutrition whom they feel they can trust.

Which Kinds of Foods Should Be Prescribed for Anorexia Nervosa Patients?

Some therapists allow a completely free choice of food, often permitting the patient to bring food into the hospital to supplement or substitute what is provided. Another approach is to use totally artificial methods of refeeding, by parenteral nutrition[9] or gastric tube feeds.[10] A third alternative is to give a high energy, nutritionally complete liquid to be drunk throughout the day, and the fourth choice is to prescribe daily meals made up of normal, everyday foods, either to supply the total energy input, or in combination with high energy drinks. The dangers inherent in permitting a free selection of food are that the patients fail to expand their very limited choice of foods, or else they may go to the other extreme and overeat, sometimes to 'binge' proportions, in order to eat their way out of hospital.[11]

If patients are to return to a healthy, varied diet, they need to learn to eat normal, everyday food within some sort of regular meal pattern, and preferably from the commencement of treatment to avoid a difficult transition at a later stage. If totally, or even predominantly, artificial foods are used to produce weight gain, patients will not experience the large amounts of real food that are necessary to put on weight, and this may reinforce the belief, commonly held by patients with anorexia nervosa, that they will gain weight on less amounts of food than those on which other people maintain weight. They will also have to endure monotonous flavoured liquids or suffer the discomfort and possible trauma of a canula or naso-gastric tube.[12] The advantages of these artificial methods of refeeding are that cooperation is not required to achieve weight gain, the energy input can be calculated accurately and the patient is spared gastric discomfort during weight gain. However, in our experience, it is quite possible to use normal food from the commencement of treatment for every patient, including the most emaciated or intransigent individual. Also, good estimates of energy intake can be made from daily prescribed menus and nurses' notes from supervised meals. Gastric discomfort can be kept to a minimum by gradually increasing the size of the diet, with the addition of high energy liquid supplements when the diet becomes excessively bulky.

From these considerations and experiences, the following protocol for refeeding patients within a hospital setting has been developed.

On admission to hospital, a daily eating plan is organized for individual patients to give a weekly weight gain of 1.5kg.[13] This can require between 6300 kilojoules and 19 000 kilojoules daily depending on the stage of weight gain, the size of the patient, their metabolic rate and their level of activity. For example, an individual who has been eating minimally before admission to hospital should initially be given a relatively small diet of around 6300 kilojoules daily. The gastric discomfort of a larger food intake would be hard to tolerate, and is unnecessary as long as such a person starts to regain weight on a small diet.

Daily menus are written for each patient by the dietitian to ensure that a variety of foods are eaten, and that each individual has an adequate energy intake. The prescribed amount of food is gradually increased, following regular discussions between the dietitian and patient, to ensure a 1.5kg weekly increase. After a few weeks of consistent weight gain, patients are allowed to start selecting their own food.

Patients are given a nutritionally balanced diet of normal hospital meals, including some high energy foods such as cake, chocolate and chips. They are not permitted to bring their own food or drink into hospital. We do not allow patients to hoard food and challenge their belief that they need 'special' foods. Commercial dietary products, such as saccharine and low fat milk products, are also forbidden as they are totally counterproductive for weight gain.

Patients with anorexia nervosa usually complain of constipation. Laxative abuse is a common occurrence and is often consumed in the form of unprocessed bran which has the added attraction in being a bulky, non-calorific food substitute. Constipation is usually the result of minimal food residue passing through the digestive system, and a diet providing fibre in the form of wholegrain cereals, fruit and vegetables will regularize most bowels. For this reason, no laxatives are allowed.

During the period of weight gain, patients' meals are supervised by nursing staff in the dining room. This is to ensure that the prescribed diet is being adhered to and to observe the patients' eating behaviour as well as setting an example of normal eating behaviour. Weekly interviews with the dietitian focus on the rate of weight gain, general eating behaviour and any fears and difficulties still being experienced by the patient. Patients are encouraged to eat the full prescribed diet but there is no form of forced feeding. Encouragement and reassurance from other patients as well as the multidisciplinary team members are usually sufficient to promote a satisfactory rate of weight gain. However, if patients fail to gain weight, they must be restricted to bed until the required weekly weight gain is achieved.[13] This restriction of activity helps them to gain weight, but also provides a strong motivation to eat their meals. If food is continually left on the plate, we encourage the individual to eat it all rather than prescribing additional food[14] as over-prescription of food will only result in more of this behaviour.

On reaching target weight, patients select all their own food, gradually reducing their daily input under supervision of the dietitian, until their weight stabilizes. This procedure can take up to 2 weeks and cannot be hurried as the weight gained is very labile and easily lost. Their final maintenance requirements can be a useful indication of the appropriateness of the target weight, and of their continued level of activity. The expected range of energy intake to maintain the typical female teenage patients at a healthy weight is between 7500 kilojoules and 10500 kilojoules daily. Therefore, if a maintenance intake is found to be less than 7500 kilojoules, the target weight is probably too low; if the energy intake at target weight is much in excess of 10500 kilojoules then the patient is likely to be doing too much exercise.[15]

Patients are supervised but to a lesser extent once they have reached their target weight and are required to keep a daily food diary. These measures are included to ensure that the size of meals and the variety of foods eaten are satisfactory. This maintenance period can be a very difficult time for many individuals. They no longer have the security of having to gain weight, and often begin to restrict their food choices for fear of over-shooting their target weight.

Patients are encouraged to stay in hospital for a few weeks after target weight is reached[16] to gain confidence in controlling their own weight maintenance, and to practise eating different foods in a variety of environments. They are encouraged to eat at home and in restaurants, and they are also challenged with occasional set meals, special cakes for afternoon tea, barbecues and other social eating situations they are likely to encounter in everyday life.

Family Counselling

Most patients regain weight without great difficulty in hospital and maintain their weight on a very sensible diet. However, their eating behaviour often deteriorates on their return home with a subsequent loss of weight. One factor in this regression is the continuing friction between the patients and their families over food and meals. Patients often anticipate close observation and interference from their parents or spouse, pressuring them to eat far more or more often than is necessary. The families usually are very anxious about the return of the patient, and unsure of how to react with the result that they often over-supervise the patient's eating.

The dietitian can defuse this situation by counselling the patient and family concerning their respective fears and uncertainties and to discuss the strategies that could be adopted to overcome them. These family sessions need to take place before discharge. However, they are also of great value a week or two after the patient has been discharged so that difficulties which have become apparent can be resolved.

Outpatient Care

Patients who are sufficiently motivated to change their eating behaviour may do so without the need of hospital admission. They are referred to the dietitian for a detailed diet history, in order to provide a structured eating pattern for weight gain. Prescribed energy intakes are graded, as for the inpatient, according to the stage and current rate of weight gain, the size of the patient, metabolic rate and level of activity. However, a lower weekly weight gain is expected because of the additional energy expenditure at school or work, and the impracticality of someone with these commitments eating a very large diet.

Meal plans are organized on an individual basis, to suit individual life styles, aiming at a weekly weight gain of around 0.5kg.

Regular sessions are held to discuss changes in the diet, to monitor the variety of foods that are being eaten, and to advise the patient about reducing food intake once target weight is reached.

There is a danger that outpatients can become dependent on the dietitian as someone to talk to endlessly about food, without necessarily increasing their weight or improving their eating habits. Patients need to talk about their food fears and can benefit from professional advice and guidance, but the dietitian has to avoid inadvertently reinforcing their obsessional behaviours and making it easier for them to maintain the status quo by making continued sessions contingent on some progress.

Nutritional Education

Nutritional education is given throughout the treatment of inpatients and out-patients, mainly in an informal fashion, answering nutritional questions as they arise and relating recommended nutritional guidelines[17] to the food that the patients are eating.

One of the most challenging aspects of the nutritional education that needs to be given is to guide the patients back to 'normal' eating. There is a danger that the patient with anorexia nervosa will merely substitute the dietitians 'diet' for all the other diets they have followed previously. This will certainly provide a healthier nutritional intake, but there is little virtue in exchanging one ritualistic eating pattern for another. It is therefore essential, if patients are to cope with the many, varied and often unpredictable eating situations that occur in everyday life, that they learn to eat in a spontaneous fashion. They also need to develop cues for eating that most people follow, such as hunger, time of day, social situation, and visual attraction. After many months, sometimes years, of eating according to their morning weight or to a very rigid meal plan, patients seem to experience great difficulty in relinquishing all the restrictions and habits they have developed. Many sessions are spent discussing this transition from restricted to relaxed eating, and patients are encouraged to experiment whilst still in the supportive and secure atmosphere of the hospital.

The dietitian has to decide what is 'normal', 'nutritious', and 'socially acceptable', all terms that have been used here but which are difficult to define. Energy and nutrient intakes have been recommended for the 'normal' population,[17] but are these appropriate for the individual who has recently lost and regained large amounts of weight?

What is a 'nutritious' food intake? The dietitian, accustomed to advising overweight, diabetic or atheroschlerotic patients, can reinforce some of the unnecessarily purist ideas that patients with anorexia nervosa have picked up from magazines, 'health food' books and media interviews. As promoters of 'good' eating, dietitians need to have a balanced view of what is healthy with what is fun to eat and practical in social situations. The Dietary Guidelines for Australia[18] include recommendations for reduced sugar and fat intakes, and more dietary fibre and the response from the general public has been so positive that food manufacturers have changed their products accordingly and promote them as such. This is to be applauded, but there is a danger that the recommendations can be misinterpreted or taken to extremes so that people can believe, for instance, that skimmed milk is always preferable to whole milk, any sugar in the diet is bad and that unprocessed bran is necessary to avoid constipation.

Along the same continuum is promotion of vitamin and mineral supplements as necessary for complete health, whereas they can be health-damaging if taken in excess. Patients often use these distorted health messages in defence of their beliefs and practices, but will listen to a different point of view put forward by a nutritionist, and with more credence than they would give to their parents or doctor advising them about diet.

Considerations of what are 'normal' and 'socially acceptable' eating habits are also very difficult, since a certain behaviour in isolation can be 'normal' whereas when taken to extremes it becomes abnormal. Unacceptable eating habits fall into 2 categories. The first is obsessional behaviour which is relatively easy to recognize and to explain to the patient as being so. Examples of this would be: eating with the same cutlery at every meal (usually the smallest utensils available), eating food on the plate in a set order, and cutting food into tiny mouthfuls. The other category is harder to define and it is sometimes only when patients are doing the same thing as a group that the behaviour stands out as being abnormal. Examples of this type of behaviour would be: making sandwiches at every meal, adding excess spice and seasoning to food, or making inappropriate mixtures.

Although seemingly trivial behaviours individually are often ignored in treatment programmes, they can represent the last vestiges of anorexia nervosa that a patient clings to in the face of imposed weight gain and dietary control, and as such could be used as indicators of poor prognosis, if maintained throughout treatment.

Summary

The dietitian, as nutritional counsellor in the treatment of anorexia nervosa, provides detailed nutritional and dietary behavioural information for the assessment and general management of patients with anorexia nervosa. The dietitian supervises the dietary management of weight gain and maintenance, provides professional guidelines for healthy, sensible eating habits and counsels families and patients for the transition from hospital meals to eating at home.

References

1. Russell, G.F.M.: General management of anorexia nervosa and difficulties in assessing the efficiacy of treatment; in Vigersky (Ed.) Anorexia Nervosa pp.277-89 (Raven Press, New York 1977)
2. Beumont, P.J.V., Chambers, T.L., Rouse L. and Abrahams, S.F.: The diet composition and nutritional knowledge of patients with anorexia nervosa. Journal of Human Nutrition, 35:265-73 (1981)
3. Chambers, T.L., Beumont, P.J.V. and Abraham, S.F.: The diet histories and nutrient intakes of anorexia nervosa patients. Food and Nutrition Notes and Reviews, 36(2):64-5 (1979).
4. Marshall, M.H.: Anorexia nervosa: dietary treatment and re-establishment of body weight in 20 cases studied on a metabolic unit. Journal of Human Nutrition 32:349-57 (1978).
5. Touyz, S.W. and Beumont, P.J.V.: The use of multimodal therapy in the treatment of anorexia nervosa. The Australian Clinical Psychologist 16(1):23-32 (1984).

6. Touyz, S.W. and Beumont, P.J.V.: Anorexia nervosa: a follow-up investigation. *The Medical Journal of Australia* 141(4): 219-22 (1984).
7. Pertschuk, M.J.: Behaviour therapy: extended follow-up; in Vigersky (Ed.) *Anorexia Nervosa*. pp.305-13 (Raven Press, New York 1977).
8. Touyz, S.W. and Beumont, P.J.V.: The use of videotape recordings in improving abnormal eating behaviour in patients with anorexia nervosa. *Proceedings of the Australian Society for Psychiatric Research* Melbourne (Abstract) (1983).
9. Pertschuk, M.J., Forster, J., Buzby, G. and Mullen, J.L.: The treatment of anorexia nervosa with total parenteral nutrition. *Biological Psychiatry* 16(6):539-50 (1981).
10. Garrow, J.S.: Dietary management of obesity and anorexia nervosa. *Journal of Human Nutrition* 34:131-8 (1980).
11. Bruch, H.: Perils of behaviour modification in treatment of anorexia nervosa. *Journal of The American Medical Association* 230: 1419-22 (1974).
12. Dally, P., Gomez, J. and Isaacs, A.J.: *Anorexia Nervosa*. (William Heinemann Medical Books Ltd., London 1979).
13. Touyz, S.W., Beumont, P.J.V., Glaun, D., Philips, T. and Cowie, I.: Comparison of a lenient and strict operant conditioning programme in refeeding patients with anorexia nervosa. *British Journal of Psychiatry* 144:512-20 (1984).
14. Agras, S. and Werne, J.: Behaviour modification in anorexia nervosa: Research Foundations; in Vigersky (Ed.) *Anorexia nervosa*. pp.291-303 (Raven Press, New York 1977).
15. Beumont, P.J.V. Hook, S. and Touyz, S.W.: Excessive exercise in anorexia nervosa. *Proceedings of the International Conference on Anorexia Nervosa and Related Diseases*. (University College, Swansea (Abstract) 1984).
16. Garfinkel, P.E. and Garner, D.M.: *Anorexia Nervosa: A Multidimensional Perspective*. (Brunner Mazel, New York 1982).
17. Truswell, A.S.: Disorders related to nutrition in the Australian community. *Food and Nutrition Notes and Reviews* 36(3): 94-9 (1979).
18. National Health and Medical Research Council *Dietary allowances for use in Australia (with explanatory notes)*. Australian Government Publishing Service, Canberra 1979.

Chapter IV

What Constitutes Recovery in Anorexia Nervosa?

There have been a number of recent reviews of outcome studies of anorexia nervosa,[1-4] all of which emphasize the importance of satisfactory diagnostic criteria, patient selection, adequate length of follow-up and the use of standardized outcome measures. However, the problem of the validity of outcome measures is not often addressed.

Garfinkel and Garner,[1] in discussing the diagnostic criteria for anorexia nervosa, favour the Pathology of Eating Group's[5] definition as the most appropriate and clinically applicable. All 3 factors must be present:

1. Self-inflicted severe loss of weight, using 1 or more of the following devices: a) avoidance of foods considered to be 'fattening' (especially carbohydrate-containing foods); b) self-induced vomiting; c) abuse of purgatives; and d) excessive exercise.

2. A secondary endocrine disorder of the hypothalamic anterior pituitary gonadal axis manifest in the female as amenorrhoea and in the male by a diminution of sexual interest and activity.

3. A psychological disorder that has as its central theme a morbid fear of being unable to control eating and hence becoming too fat.

While this definition, as Yager[6] comments, is deficient for research purposes as it does not define the amount of weight loss, it contains the 3 features of weight, endocrine disorder and attitude towards eating and fatness that need to be addressed in a discussion of recovery from the syndrome.

A former sufferer could be said to be recovered if they are stably at normal weight, have normal endocrine functioning and no abnormal eating behaviour or fear of fatness. The word 'recovered' is not used in this sense in the majority of outcome studies. Not infrequently, the criteria for recovery are not stated clearly. Hsu,[3] in reviewing 16 outcome studies in which the diagnostic criteria were satisfactory, there were at least 15 subjects and the mean follow-up time was at least 2 years, found that half of the studies had an inadequate definition of what is 'normal', 'cured' and 'recovered'. Steinhausen and Glanville, [4] reporting on 45 follow-up studies (including the 16 reported on by Hsu), found that in 15 of the 45 studies, the percentage of average weight was not documented, in 14 menstruation was not documented, and in 17 no disordered eating behaviour was documented. Only 40% of the studies had documented all 3 factors. Many of these studies are nevertheless used as evidence for treatment success and for prognostic factors.

Standardized Outcome Measures

None of the published outcome measures requires recovery to be in all 3 areas of weight, endocrine functioning and eating disorder signs and symptoms. The most accepted outcome measures are those designed by Morgan and Russell[7] for use in long-term outpatient follow-up of 41 patients and more recently Morgan et al. have used the same measures for follow-up of 78 consecutively presenting patients at Bristol.[8] These measures have also been used by Hsu et al.[9] and in a modified form by others.[10-12] There are 2 measures of outcome

1. The 3-category 'general outcome' is based solely on weight and menstruation. A 'good' outcome is weight stable within 15% of average for age and height and regular menstruation for the 6 months before follow-up. 'Intermediate' outcome is weight not stable within 15% average, and/or irregular menstruation. 'Poor' outcome is persistent low weight with absent menstruation.

2. The global outcome score, named 'the average outcome score', is based on a semi-structured interview. Ten per cent of the score measures weight, 10% 'reduction of food intake', 20% menstruation, 20% sexual adjustment, 20% mental state, and 20% social and vocational adjustment.

Another global score is that devised by Garfinkel et al.[13] for use in follow-up of 42 inpatients and subsequently used by Vandereycken and Pierloot.[14] In this score, eating disorder behaviour forms half of the score with equal weighting being given to food faddism, vomiting, bingeing and laxative abuse. Menstruation forms less than 10% of the score, weight less than 15%, and less than 20% is formed from social and vocational scales. The authors categorize the patient's state as 'excellent' when the score is less than 5 out of a possible 23 points and patients who are amenorrhoeric would be categorized as having an 'excellent' recovery provided they were virtually free from other signs and symptoms.

Weight

Weight is the only objective measurement of recovery, provided it is measured. There are, however, considerable difficulties defining 'normal' weight. The commonest solution adopted is to use the Metropolitan Life Insurance figures produced in 1959 in the USA for average weight for age and height for insured persons over the age of 15[15] and to define 'normal' as a weight within either 10% or 15% of average. The problem of 'normal' weight for age and height is greater for children, and there are also considerable problems in assessing 'normal' weight for adolescent males who complete skeletal growth later than females and whose percentage of weight as body fat is less.[16]

Endocrine Functioning

Whether or not the endocrine dysfunction in anorexia nervosa is a secondary symptom of the syndrome is still an unanswered question [17] and in order to clarify this it is important that endocrine function is as fully documented as possible at follow-up.

Menstruation

The degree of irregularity of the menses which is considered normal is usually not stated in follow-up studies. In Morgan's categories irregularity of menstruation by itself categorizes the patient as having an 'intermediate' outcome rather than a 'good' outcome. Although return of menstruation is significantly related to weight in all studies, the overall figures conceal individual differences. There is insufficient information from studies of anorexia nervosa patients at long-term follow-up to support a hypothesis that the patient needs to attain approximately 20% of bodyweight in fat to resume regular menstruation as has been shown to be the case with the onset of menarche.[16] It is possible that there is a difference in sensitivity of the complex mechanism of the hypothalamic pituitary axis to factors like bodyweight in older women compared with adolescent girls. The objections to excluding amenorrhoea in females as a diagnostic criterion for anorexia nervosa outlined by Halmi [18] apply to excluding return of menstruation as a criterion for recovery.

Normal menstruation cannot be assessed when the patient is taking a contraceptive hormone.

Sexual Functioning

For both male and female patients, data should be collected on fertility, libido and sexual performance. Morgan's sexual adjustment scale estimates attitudes towards sexuality and sexual behaviour on 4 sub-scales. The highest aim for sexual relationships – 'marriage with children' – has an old-fashioned ring! Male patients should be specifically asked about return of spontaneous erections and beard growth.

The varying age range of anorexia nervosa patients at follow-up makes the estimation of 'normal' sexual attitudes and behaviour difficult. In humans the relationship between sexual attitudes and behaviour and hypothalamic pituitary gonadal axis functioning is complex, and sexual behaviour is probably at least as much influenced by social factors as hormonal levels.

Eating Behaviour and Fear of Fatness

Behaviour such as food restriction, type and quantity of food, pattern of eating, purging behaviour and exercise aimed at weight reduction, as well as attitudes to food and weight and body size need to be documented. The assessment of these behaviours in a follow-up situation is dependent on patient cooperation. Theander [19] found that the sympathetic and knowledgeable interviewer could obtain good patient cooperation in revealing abnormal behaviour and attitudes. Although it is desirable, as suggested by Steinhausen and Glanville,[4] that accounts from relatives and friends should be sought, this should be regarded as an adjunct to the patient's account, as abnormal behaviours and attitudes are often concealed from relatives and friends. Recently developed scales such as the Eating Attitudes Test[20] and the Eating Disorder Inventory[21] will be useful adjuncts to clinical interviews of patients at follow-up. A standardized semi-structured interview for eliciting eating disorder symptoms would be a useful tool for follow-up. Most investigators have given few details of how eating disorder symptoms were elicited.[13, 14, 22, 23]

Other Features

The 2 global assessment scores both have sub-scales measuring personal relationships and vocational functioning, and Morgan's score has a sub-scale for mental state. Symptoms in these areas are not part of the diagnostic criteria for the syndrome used in most research, [24-27] but because it is suspected that the anorexia nervosa syndrome may reflect developmental and emotional difficulties, full assessment of the patient's personality, social functioning and psychiatric symptomatology at follow-up is desirable. This would be better recorded separately from recovery from the syndrome itself. Halmi [18] has suggested a multi-axial method of diagnosis for anorexia nervosa and this would be a useful way of recording findings at follow-up.

The ideal outcome assessment would be by standardized semi-structured interview by an independent interviewer knowledgeable about the condition, and recording weight, menstruation, sexual functioning and eating disorder behaviours and attitudes as well as psychiatric symptoms and life functioning. Information from relatives and friends should desirably be obtained, particularly as state over the preceding year rather than just in the interview situation needs to be estimated. Such an interview needs to be supplemented by self-administered questionnaires such as the EAT and the EDI.

The follow-up should be at a minimum of 4 years although this time is inadequate to assess hormonal functioning in some patients and also inadequate to assess life functioning in younger patients. Theander, whose original follow-up of 94 patients was at a minimum of 6 years, [19] found some patients were still improving and his further follow-up 16 years later confirmed this and also the poor prognosis for unrecovered patients, the death rate for the whole series having risen to 18%.[28]

Outcome Study of 46 Female Patients with Anorexia Nervosa

The practical difficulties of defining 'recovery' are illustrated from a follow-up study of 50 consecutively presenting female patients with anorexia nervosa fulfilling Feighner criteria.[24] They were followed up at a minimum of 4 years (mean 8 years) from onset of amenorrhoea and a minimum of 3.9 years from presentation. They had been treated for a mean of 2.5 years by the author. The mean age at onset was 16.2 years (S.D. ± 2.7) and mean age at follow-up was 25.7 years (S.D. ± 6.7). All patients were traced but full data was only obtained on 46 patients (92%), 3 by written information from overseas patients, and 43 by interview. The interview was conducted by an independent psychiatrist familiar with anorexia nervosa. In addition to measurement of height and weight and Morgan's semi-structured interview, particular attention was paid to the eliciting of eating disorder symptoms and psychiatric symptomatology. The main aims of the study were to identify patients who were completely healthy and to relate eating disorder symptoms to psychiatric state. This study is described in detail elsewhere.[29] A further aim was to assess the relationship of Morgan's outcome categories based on weight and menstruation to eating disorder symptoms, and the results of this part of the study are presented here.

Weight

All weights were converted to a percentage of average weight for age and height.[15] The relationship of percentage weight to menstruation and eating disorder signs and symptoms are shown in figures 4.1 and 4.2.

Low Weight

Of the 47 patients whose weights were known at follow-up, 17 were below 85% of average weight. All of them fulfilled one of the diagnostic criteria of anorexia nervosa of DSM 111[25] 'refusal to maintain bodyweight over a minimal normal

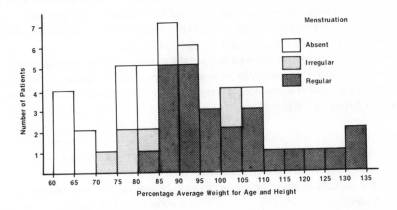

Fig. 4.1 Relationship of menstruation to weight at follow-up (47 patients)

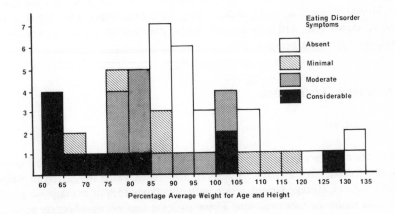

Fig. 4.2 Relationship of eating disorder symptoms to weight at follow-up (46 patients)

weight for age and height'. While in 13 patients this low weight was associated with a restricted lifestyle because of at least moderate anorexic type symptoms and behaviour; 4 patients merit comment. One 30-year-old career woman had minimal food and weight concern and was primarily handicapped by a recurrent severe major depressive disorder.[25] In such a patient it is difficult to estimate the interrelationship of low weight and depressive illness. One patient was happily married and highly effective in her career and personal and social relationships and had adjusted to her restrictive eating habits and weight phobia to the point where they interfered very little with her life. One patient, after 14 years of anorexia nervosa, was losing her eating disorder symptoms and after the formal follow-up had a much-wanted normal pregnancy. One patient who was happily breast-feeding a six-month-old child considered herself to be recovered from her anorexia nervosa. However, ovulation had been induced hormonally by her gynaecologist, and her failure to gain weight during pregnancy, weight loss during breast-feeding (76% of average weight for age and height at age 27), together with the fact that she had never allowed her weight to reach 90% of average and had never menstruated spontaneously in the 10 years since her onset of anorexia nervosa, would suggest a continuing weight phobia. Her life was, however, in all respects a happy and fulfilled one.

Obesity

Five patients were more than 15% above average weight for age and height. One was intensely and continuously concerned with food and weight, but the other 4 patients, all with onset of anorexia nervosa before age 15, were in their late teens, plump, attractive, well proportioned girls who had gained weight by overeating during the recovery phase more than a year previously and had been at a stable weight since and were not concerned enough about weight to diet. They were all functioning well in all aspects of their lives. They did not qualify for Morgan's 'good' category because they were overweight although they considered themselves, and were considered by the interviewer, to have recovered from their anorexia nervosa.

Endocrine Dysfunction

Menstruation

Restoration of menstruation was related to weight as can be seen in figure 1. However, 3 patients, all over 25 years of age, menstruated irregularly at weights below 80% of average weight. Four patients above 85% of average weight had not had return of menstruation. These patients had no significantly abnormal eating habits or concerns about weight. No pattern emerged from study of the individual details of the 4 patients. Two of them, with onset respectively at 14 and 19 years, had had 4 years of severe food restriction but had eaten normally for the preceding year and weight was still increasing slowly. One 25-year-old patient had had only 3 slight menstrual bleeds during 3 years of weight over 90% of average and a happy well-adjusted life. Before the sudden onset of severe anorexia nervosa at age 18, she had menstruated only occasionally although she had been at normal weight with no dietary restrictions or athletic involvement. One patient in the past history of her anorexia nervosa had had return of menstruation for several months shortly after a rapid inpatient restoration to average weight, had become amenorrhoeic with subsequent weight loss, but when weight reached and passed average weight more slowly as an outpatient, menstruation had not resumed despite a stable weight of 110% of average for a year.

Sexual Functioning

Fertility

Eight patients had had children since onset of their anorexia nervosa, but this was no guarantee of recovery. Only 3 of the 8 patients had become pregnant when fully recovered from their syndromes. Two patients who were below 85% average weight at follow-up were parous. One of them has already been discussed as a low-weight patient. One 35-year-old binge-vomiter had 7 years previously allowed her weight to rise sufficiently for her to become pregnant, maintained weight during pregnancy and breast-feeding, and then resumed her symptomatology. Two normal-weight binge-vomiting patients' symptoms had been unchanged by childbirth. One patient had been originally referred post-partum for laxative abuse which had been present, together with bulimia, since shortly after the onset of anorexia nervosa at 14 years of age.

Sexual Responsiveness

The ability to have orgasm was also not closely related to other features, and one amenorrhoeic patient at 82% of average weight stated that she was orgasmic in a sexual relationship with her boyfriend, although in addition to being underweight, she suffered from binge-vomiting and continual weight preoccupation.

The life situation for patients at follow-up, the majority of whom were in their twenties, was markedly different from the presentation of adolescent girls at the onset of their anorexia nervosa. Only 16 patients had not had sexual intercourse. Eight of these were over the age of 20, and 7 actively avoided sexual relationships but were also inhibited in relationships in other ways. Eight were under 21 years, and 6 either had boyfriends or wished to have one and/or looked forward to sexual involvement in the future. As has been shown in other studies, [30, 31] patients with anorexia nervosa do not necessarily differ from their contemporaries in their sexual attitudes and behaviour.

Males did not form part of this follow-up study, but in the 9 male patients currently being followed up there are the same difficulties in assessment in that sexual behaviour is variable during and after recovery and appears to be at least as much influenced by cultural and personal factors as hormonal ones.

Assessment of Eating Disorder Symptoms

Eliciting of eating disorder symptoms can be extremely difficult in newly presenting anorexia nervosa patients who are resentful about their referral and treatment. This was not found to be the case in the follow-up interviews. The 43 patients who attended for the 3- to 4-hour interview initially filled in a set of questionnaires, 1 of which was based on Morgan's semi-structured interview. Subsequently, after rapport had been established with the independent interviewer by discussion of their general life situation and state of health and well-being, patients were systematically questioned not only about vomiting, bingeing and laxative abuse, but about their daily diet, carbohydrate and fat avoidance, calorie consciousness, eating with others, and frequency of weighing and exercising. After the formal follow-up interview they were further assessed by the author who had been responsible for their treatment.

For the first 12 patients parents were interviewed separately but subsequently parents were not formally interviewed as the patients revealed far more about themselves and their behaviour than was known to their parents. The 3 overseas patients who gave full information about themselves all admitted readily to considerable food-weight preoccupations.

On the basis of the combined information about eating and weight concerns and behaviour, patients were assigned to 1 of 4 categories of eating disorder symptoms, 1. nil; 2. minimal; 3. moderate; 4. considerable to continuous.
Nil: 15 patients had no eating disorder symptoms. They ate a full range of foods without anxiety, had lost their knowledge of kilojoules, and accepted their body size realistically. Typical of these patients were comments like 'I used to know the calorie content of every food but now I can't be bothered with that sort of thing', 'It is such a relief not worrying about food and weight – I can hardly believe that I used to be like that'. Of particular note in these patients was the absence of self-critical comments about their appearance, which had been so prominent during their illness.
Mild: 8 patients during the preceding 6 months had had fleeting concerns about weight and eating or were mildly diet-conscious *or* had no more than 2 episodes of mild binge-eating but no purging behaviour or excessive exercising. These patients considered themselves and were considered by both interviewers to be recovered from the 'fear of being unable to control eating and hence becoming too fat'.

Table 1. Relationship of general outcome to eating disorder symptom (46 patients).

Eating disorder symptoms	Morgan's general outcome category		
	'Good'	'Intermediate'	'Poor'
Nil	9	6	0
Mild	3	4	1
Moderate	3	5	4
Considerable	0	4	7
Total	15	19	12

Moderate: 12 patients had food-weight preoccupation and/or bingeing and/or purging that occurred more than occasionally, but less than half of their time was taken up with eating disorder symptoms.
Considerable: 11 patients had at least half their time taken up with weight and eating concerns or behaviour irrespective of the amount of improvement in these symptoms and behaviours compared with their state at presentation.

Relationship of Morgan's General Outcome Category to 'Recovery'

Table 1 shows the relationship of the general outcome categories based solely on weight and menstruation to the degree of eating disorder symptoms. If 'nil' and 'mild' are taken to mean essentially recovered from eating disorder symptoms, only 3 patients in the 'good' category retained significant symptoms. Conversely, in the 'poor' category all patients except 1 (the patient suffering from major depressive disorder) had significant eating disorder symptoms. In the 'intermediate' category 10 patients (approximately 50%) had no significant eating disorder symptoms. They were in the category because of menstrual abnormality (4), overweight (4), and weight not stable within 15% of average in the preceding 6 months (2).

Alternative Outcome Categories

The patients were further categorized into a 3-category outcome based solely on weight and eating disorder symptoms.
'Recovered': 19 patients were at stable weight above a minimal normal weight

Table 2. Alternative outcome category (46 patients). Morgan's general outcome category in parentheses.

Recovered*	Weight Recovered†	Not recovered†
(12 'good')	(3 'good')	(5 'int')
19	10	17
(7 'int')	(7 'int')	(12 'poor')

* Stable weight above 85% average more than one year.
  Nil or minimal eating disorder symptoms.
† Weight above 85% average more than one year.
  More than minimal eating disorder symptoms.

(85% of average) for over 1 year and absence or virtual absence of eating disorder symptoms.

'Weight Recovered': In 10 patients low weight was not a problem (above 85% of average weight over 1 year) but significant eating disorder symptoms were present.

'Not Recovered': 17 patients remained at low weight or weight gain was so recent that recovery could not be assured. Table 2 shows the results of this alternative outcome category with the results of Morgan's categories based on weight and menstruation in brackets.

How Should Recovery Be Categorized?

Morgan's categories based on weight and menstruation are satisfactorily standardized measures. They are simple to apply and relatively few patients in the 'good' category of stable normal weight and menstruation have other eating disorder symptoms to a significant degree.

Although in this study a few overweight adolescent patients were apparently recovered in other respects, in general, in a disorder where weight and eating abnormalities are a central feature, normalization of weight (within 15% of average) should continue to be a requirement for a good outcome.

Endocrine disorder is also a diagnostic feature and normalization of menstruation in the female and sexual function in the male should also be required for outcome to be categorized as 'good'.

The 'good' outcome category should also require that the patient be free of other eating disorder symptoms. The difficulty with this requirement is the lack of a simply applied standardized method of proven validity. When sufficient experience has been accumulated from the use of questionnaires such as the EAT and the EDI at long-term follow-up of patients with anorexia nervosa, it may be valid to exclude from the 'good' category any patient who scores above an agreed maximum, say 20 points, on the EAT. Currently clinical assessment is essential and is best done by standardized semi-structured interview conducted by an independent experienced interviewer thoroughly familiar with the disorder. One format for grading the results of such an interview has been outlined. Psychiatric symptoms other than eating disorder symptoms should be recorded separately. [29]

All reports of long-term outcome studies of anorexia nervosa identify a minimum of approximately 20% of patients who remain severely handicapped.[8] Because of the deficiencies in the outcome measures currently being used, it is not known what proportion of patients in the various published series are fully recovered from the syndrome.

For identification of prognostic factors and evaluation of treatment methods any category of 'good', 'normal', 'cured' or 'recovered' should include only patients who are at stable weight within 15% of average, have normal gonadal functioning, and have no more than minimal eating disorder symptoms.

References

1. Garfinkel, P.E. and Garner, D.M.: *Anorexia Nervosa. A Multidimensional Perspective.* (Brunner/Mazel, New York 1982).
2. Schwartz, D.M. and Thompson, M.G.: Do Anorectics Get Well? Current Research and Future Needs. *American Journal of Psychiatry* 138: 319-23 (1981).
3. Hsu, L.K.G.: Outcome of Anorexia Nervosa. A Review of the Literature (1954-1978). *Archives of General Psychiatry* 37: 1041-6 (1980).
4. Steinhausen, H.C. and Glanville, K.: Follow-up Studies of Anorexia Nervosa: A Review of Research Findings. *Psychological Medicine* 13: 239-49 (1983).
5. Garrow, J.S.; Crisp, A.H.; Jordan, H.A.; Meyer, J.E.; Russell, G.F.M.; Silverstone, T.; Stunkard, A.J. and Van Itallie, T.B.: Pathology of Eating, group report; in Silverstone (Ed) *Dahlen Konferenzen Life Sciences Research Report* 2, Berlin (1975).
6. Yager, J.: Book Review. *International Journal of Eating Disorders* 2(4): 243-8 (1983).
7. Morgan, H.G. and Russell, G.F.M.: Value of family background and clinical features as predictors of long-term outcome in anorexia nervosa: four-year follow-up study of 41 patients. *Psychological Medicine* 5: 355-71 (1975).
8. Morgan, H.G.; Purgold, J. and Welbourne, J.: Management and Outcome in Anorexia Nervosa. A Standardised Prognostic Study. *British Journal of Psychiatry* 143: 282-7 (1983).
9. Hsu, L.K.G.; Crisp, A.H. and Harding, B.: Outcome of Anorexia Nervosa *Lancet* 1: 61-5 (1979).
10. Sturzenberger, S.; Cantwell, D.P.; Burroughs, J.; Salkin, B. and Green, J.K.: A Follow-up Study of Adolescent Psychiatric Inpatients with Anorexia Nervosa. *Journal of American Academy of Child Psychiatry* 16: 703-13 (1977).
11. Goetz, P.; Succop, R.A.; Reihart, J.B. and Miller, A.: Anorexia Nervosa in Children: A Follow-up Study. *American Journal of Orthopsychiatry* 47: 597-603 (1977).

12. Steinhausen, H.C. and Glanville, K.: A Long-term Follow-up of Adolescent Anorexia Nervosa. *Acta Psychiatrica Scandinavica* 68: 1-10 (1983).

13. Garfinkel, P.E.; Moldofsky, H. and Garner, D.M.: The Outcome of Anorexia Nervosa: Significance of Clinical Features, Body Image, and Behaviour Modification; in Vigersky (Ed) *Anorexia Nervosa*. (Raven Press, New York 1977).

14. Vandereycken, W. and Pierloot, R.: The significance of subclassification in anorexia nervosa: a comparative study of clinical features in 141 patients. *Psychological Medicine* 13: 543-9 (1983).

15. Diem, K. and Lenther (Eds): *Geigy Scientific Tables* 7th Edition (Ciba-Geigy, Basel 1970).

16. Frish, R.: Nutrition Fatness Puberty and Fertility. *Comprehensive Therapy* 7: 15-23 (1981).

17. Weiner, H.: The Hypothalamic-Pituitary-Ovarian Axis in Anorexia and Bulimia Nervosa. *International Journal of Eating Disorders* 2(4): 109-16 (1983).

18. Halmi, K.: Classification of Eating Disorders. *International Journal of Eating Disorders* 2(4): 21-6 (1983).

19. Theander, S.: Anorexia Nervosa – A Psychiatric Investigation of 94 Female Cases. *Acta Psychiatrica Scandinavica* Supplementum 214 (1970).

20. Garner, D.M.; Olmsted, M.P.; Bohr, Y. and Garfinkel, P.E.: The Eating Attitudes Test: psychometric features and clinical correlates. *Psychological Medicine* 12: 871-8 (1982).

21. Garner, D.M.; Olmsted, M.P. and Polivy, J.: Development and Validation of a Multidimensional Eating Disorder Inventory for Anorexia Nervosa and Bulimia. *International Journal of Eating Disorders* 2(2): 15-34 (1983).

22. Abraham, S.F.; Mira, M. and Llewellyn-Jones, D.: Bulimia: A Study of Outcome. *International Journal of Eating Disorders* 2(4): 175-80 (1983).

23. Button, E.J. and Whitehouse, A.: Subclinical Anorexia Nervosa. *Psychological Medicine* 11: 509-16 (1981).

24. Feighner, J.P.; Robins, E.; Guze, S.B.; Woodruff, R.A.; Winokur, G. and Munoz, R.: Diagnostic Criteria for Use in Psychiatric Research. *Archives of General Psychiatry* 26: 57-63 (1972).

25. American Psychiatric Association: *Diagnostic and Statistical Manual of Mental Disorders* (3rd Ed) (Washington D.C. 1980).

26. Russell, G.F.M.: Anorexia Nervosa: Its identity as an illness and its treatment; in Price (Ed) *Modern Trends in Psychological Medicine* 2. (Butterworths, London 1970).

27. Crisp, A.H.: Some aspects of the evolution presentation and follow-up of anorexia nervosa. *Proceedings Royal Society of Medicine* 58: 814-20 (1965).

28. Theander, S.: Research on Outcome and Prognosis of Anorexia Nervosa and some results from a Swedish long-term study. *International Journal of Eating Disorders* 2(4): 167-75 (1983).

29. Hall, A.; Slim, E. and Hawker, F.: Anorexia Nervosa – Long-term outcome in 50 female patients. *British Journal of Psychiatry* 145: 407-13 (1984).

30. Abraham, S.F. and Beumont, P.J.V.: Varieties of Psychosexual Experience in Patients with Anorexia Nervosa. *International Journal of Eating Disorders* 1(3): 10-19 (1982).

31. Buvat-Herbaut, M.; Hebbinckuys, P.; Lemarie, A. and Buval, J.: Attitudes towards weight, body-image, eating, menstruations, pregnancy and sexuality in 81 cases of anorexia nervosa compared to 288 normal control school girls. *International Journal of Eating Disorders* 2(4): 45-60 (1983).

Chapter V

Are Anorexia Nervosa and Bulimia Different Entities?

There is no clear-cut quantitative evidence to suggest that the eating disorders anorexia nervosa and bulimia are separate syndromes as proposed by the American Psychiatric Association.[1] It is known that patients with eating disorders may fulfil the diagnostic criteria of both anorexia nervosa and bulimia concurrently and have features in common, such as the use of weight-losing behaviour and a menstrual disturbance.[2] This evidence supports the proposition that bulimia is a variant of anorexia nervosa, as proposed by Russell.[3] On the other hand some patients with bulimia have never attained body weights below the 'desirable' range and do not wish to.[2]

If bulimia is a separate syndrome rather than a variant of anorexia nervosa, there appears a need for a quantitative tool which can differentiate between the groups of patients, for both clinical and research purposes. The term bulimia is used to refer to the syndrome and binge-eating to the behaviour.

The aim of this chapter is to present the preliminary findings from the development of an eating disorder questionnaire in order to obtain some quantitative understanding of how patients with bulimia differ from patients with anorexia nervosa and how patients who have an eating disorder differ from people who have no disordered eating behaviour.

Methods and Subjects

The questionnaire, the Eating Visual Analogue (EVA) (appendix A), was administered to 3 groups of women. The control group consisted of 69 school and 67 university students who were chosen at random during teaching sessions: as far as could be determined none of them had been diagnosed as having bulimia or anorexia nervosa. The other 2 groups consisted of 43 patients diagnosed as having bulimia,[1] and 26 patients diagnosed as having anorexia nervosa[4] by 2 of the investigators. These 2 groups of patients were receiving treatment as outpatients. The descriptive details of the 3 groups are shown in Table 1. The women were asked to complete EVA. The instructions (appendix A) were read to each subject and they were asked to complete the example item by marking the line with a short vertical mark which crossed the horizontal line. The length of the horizontal line was 10cm and each completed item was given a score of 0 to 10 (0.5cm intervals). The extremes of scoring are shown in the appendix.

Following completion of EVA the women were also asked to complete a questionnaire which enquired about eating behaviours, bodyweight changes, weight-losing behaviours and menstrual disturbances since the age of 13 years.

The data from EVA were analysed by linear discriminate analysis and Wilks Lambda was used as criterion for judging similarity between groups.[5] The 'direct method' rather than 'stepwise analysis' was considered appropriate to form the discriminate functions, as this used all the variables. Following Klecka's suggestion[5] we used the correlations between the discriminate functions and individual variables to name the dimensions (factors). The axes were rotated using Varimax as a criterion.[6]

The items of history were used as the individual data or as group frequences where appropriate. The clinical notes for the 2 patient groups were consulted after analysis of the data.

Table 1. Descriptive details of the 3 subjects groups – anorexia nervosa, bulimia and control subjects.[8]

Group	At Study				Since age 13 years	
	Number	Age (years)	Weight (kilograms)		Percentage of Standard Bodyweight	
					highest	Lowest
Bulimia	43	24 ± 7	59 ± 8	104% ± 14%	124% ± 18%	90% ± 12%
Anorexia Nervosa	26	21 ± 8	43 ± 8	78% ± 12%	103% ± 14%	65% ± 10%
Control	1226	19 ± 5	55 ± 7	100% ± 10%	109% ± 12%	94% ± 11%

Table 2. Eating Visual Analogue (EVA). Rotated correlations between discriminant functions and discriminating variables.

Factor 1 (61% variance)			Factor II (39% variance)		
Item No.	Do you:	Correlation	Item No.	Do you:	Correlation
13	go on eating binges	0.669	8	find thoughts of food going around in your mind	0.522
5	feel you have control over how much you eat	0.427	1	think about food	0.480
6	always eat everything on your plate	0.400	11	diet	0.456
14	feel you are overweight	0.375	3	count calories	0.434
15	think that you are overweight	0.290	13	go on eating binges	0.399
19	find it difficult to control your bodyweight	0.282	12	try to control weight	0.350
			10	talk a lot about food	0.343
			2	weigh the food you eat	0.325
			7	weigh yourself	0.288

Results

All EVA items, except 16 and 9, discriminated highly (p < 0.001) between patients with anorexia nervosa, bulimia and controls. Item 16 'Do you wish to change the shape of parts of your body' was significant (p < 0.01), while item 9 'Do you collect recipes' did not discriminate between the groups.

Linear discriminate analysis produced 2 factors (dimensions). Factor I accounted for 61% of the variance and Factor II 39%. The items contained in each factor and their correlations with the factor are shown in Table 2. It appears that the items loading on Factor I relate to feelings of 'control over bodyweight and eating', while those loading on Factor II relate to 'a preoccupation with bodyweight and food'. Factor I differentiated patients with anorexia nervosa from patients with bulimia and, to a lesser extent, from controls. This suggests that patients with anorexia nervosa feel in control of their eating and bodyweight, while patients with bulimia feel out of control. Factor II differentiated patients with eating disorders from controls and, to a lesser extent, from each other. This suggests that patients with eating disorders feel more preoccupied with bodyweight and food than control subjects.

The next stage of the analysis was to discriminate functions derived from EVA to classify the women into the 3 groups and to compare this classification with the classification made on clinical criteria. Thus EVA *predicted* the diagnosis, whilst the clinical diagnosis was the *actual* diagnosis. The analysis showed an 85% agreement between the predicted and the actual diagnosis (Table 3).

The history forms were examined. Of the 10 control subjects predicted by EVA as having anorexia nervosa, 6 of the women, at some stage, had reduced their bodyweight to less than 80% of standard bodyweight and 4 had experienced episodes of amenorrhoea or oligomenorrhoea. One young woman denied dieting or other weight-losing behaviours but had been treated for amenorrhoea and weight loss at age 15. All the 10 control subjects classified by EVA as having

Table 3. Agreement between classification 'predicted' by EVA and 'actual' classification.

Group Membership 'actual'		Group membership 'predicted' by EVA					
		Bulimia		Anorexia nervosa		Control	
	n	n	%	n	%	n	%
Bulimia	43	39	91%	1	2%	3	7%
Anorexia nervosa	26	3	12%	21	81%	2	8%
Control	126	10	8%	10	8%	106	84%

bulimia, considered that 'binge-eating' was a major problem for them and although not diagnosed, 8 of them were considered as having bulimia as defined earlier. Three of the 43 patients with bulimia were classified by EVA as 'controls'. At the time of completing EVA, 2 of these women had ceased to binge-eat and the third was found to have a gross personality defect. The 1 patient with bulimia who was classified by EVA as having anorexia nervosa had a prior history of binge-eating at school and was preoccupied with her bodyweight, weight loss and food.

The 2 patients with anorexia nervosa classified by EVA as 'control' completed EVA during refeeding and have maintained their weight since that time. The 3 patients with anorexia nervosa classified by EVA as having bulimia were experiencing episodes of binge-eating more than once a week, considered their binge-eating a major problem, induced vomiting and abused laxatives.

Discussion

The use of EVA to predict an eating disorder suggests that, in agreement with the view of the American Psychiatric Association,[1] anorexia nervosa and bulimia are 2 separate diagnostic entities, rather than bulimia being a variant of anorexia nervosa. However, our data suggest that some patients with eating disorders can move from one illness to the other, and that the main quantitative difference between anorexia nervosa and bulimia is related to feelings of 'control over bodyweight and eating behaviour'. Patients with anorexia nervosa feel in control, while patients with bulimia feel out of control. Thus, a patient with anorexia nervosa may *fear* a loss of control over her bodyweight and her eating, especially if she experiences occasional episodes of binge-eating,[7] but she remains in control. If a patient with anorexia nervosa binge-eats with increasing frequency and this is not controlled by her weight-losing behaviours, she not only fears a loss of control, but *feels* out of control of her weight and eating behaviour. However, it is also probable that a patient with anorexia nervosa may become a bulimia patient without going through a phase of non-disordered eating as patients with eating disorders are quantitatively different from patients who do not have an eating disorder in terms of feeling 'preoccupied with bodyweight and food'. The more the feelings of preoccupation the more likely is the diagnosis to be an eating disorder.

The relationship between the 2 conditions, normal eating behaviours and the 2-dimensional nature of factors is shown diagramatically in figure 5.1; this also shows how patients can move from having anorexia nervosa to bulimia or to becoming 'normal' eaters.

The aim of this chapter is to present quantitative data to assist in the understanding of eating disorders, and to help clarify current contentious issues. The

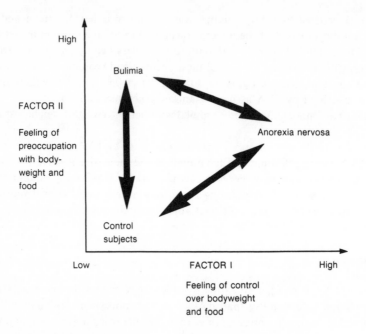

Fig. 5.1 Diagrammatic representation of the relationship between patients with anorexia nervosa, bulimia and people without eating disorders.

aim is not to present a questionnaire which is ready for use as a clinical or research tool. The very high level of agreement between classification by EVA and by clinical diagnosis, the high agreement between EVA and the history forms, the high discrimination between most of the items on EVA and the clinical sense of the factors suggest further work on EVA would be fruitful. This may enable clinicians to determine if a patient with anorexia nervosa, following refeeding, will relapse, develop bulimia or recover and similarly, if a patient with bulimia, after ceasing binge-eating, is likely to relapse, develop anorexia nervosa or recover.

References

1. American Psychiatric Association: *Diagnostic and Statistical Manual of Mental Disorders* 3rd ed. (1980).
2. Abraham, S.F. and Beumont, P.J.V.: How patients describe binge eating. *Psychological Medicine* 12: 625-35 (1982).
3. Russell, G.F.M.: Bulimia nervosa, an ominous variant of anorexia nervosa. *Psychological Medicine* 9: 429-48 (1979).

4. Russell, G.F.M.: Anorexia nervosa: its identity as an illness, and its treatment; in Prince (Ed.) *Modern Trends in Psychological Medicine* II. pp. 131-64 (Butterworths, London 1970).
5. Klecka, W.R.: *Discriminant Analysis*. (Sage Publications, London 1980).
6. Nie, N.H.; Hull, C.H.; Jenkins, J.G.; Steinbenner, K. and Bent, D.H.: *The Statistical Package for the Social Sciences* 2nd ed. p. 485 (McGraw Hill, New York 1975).
7. Feighner, J.; Robins, E.; Guse, S.; Woodruft, R.A.; Winoker, G. and Munoz, R.: Diagnostic criteria for use in psychiatric research. *Archives of General Psychiatry* 26: 57-63 (1972).
8. Diem, K. (Ed): *Geigy Scientific Tables*, 6th ed. Geigy Pharmaceuticals, St. Leonards, NSW 559: 615-22 (1962).

Chapter VI

The Prevalence of Bulimia in an Australian University Sample

Over the last decade there has been an increased concern among women in contemporary society to maintain a slim figure. This concern has been associated with a rapid growth in gymnasia and fad diets as well as a boom in the health food industry. Schwartz *et al.* have even suggested that the current emphasis on diet and exercise has 'shifted from a growing leisure time hobby to a national obsession'.[1] The anxiety regarding the maintenance of a desirable bodyweight and shape has been accompanied by an increased prevalence of eating disorders such as anorexia nervosa and more recently bulimia [1-7].

Bulimia is an eating disorder which occurs primarily in young women and is characterized by recurrent episodes of gorging or binge-eating.[8] These episodes are usually followed by feelings of guilt and remorse at the loss of self-control and acute anxiety regarding the possibility of gaining unwanted weight.[5] Patients usually begin a stringent diet, induce vomiting or abuse purgatives to normalise their weight after an episode of binge-eating. The diagnostic criteria for bulimia are presented in Table 1.

Binge-eating has been described in obese individuals [9,10] as well as in a subgroup of patients with anorexia nervosa.[11-14] There have been several recent reports in the literature suggesting that the incidence of bulimia in normal-weight young women has increased dramatically.[5,15-22] The prevalence of bulimia has recently been estimated to be as high as 20% among female university students in the United States.[23]

Table 1. Criteria for diagnosis of bulimia.

A. Recurrent episodes of binge-eating (rapid consumption of a large amount of food in a discrete period of time, usually less than 2 hours)

B. At least 3 of the following:
1. consumption of high caloric, easily ingested food during a binge;
2. inconspicuous eating during a binge;
3. termination of such eating episodes by abdominal pain, sleep, social interruption or self-induced vomiting;
4. repeated attempts to lose weight by severely restrictive diets, self-induced vomiting or use of cathartics and/or diuretics.
5. frequent weight fluctuations greater than 4.5kg due to alternating binges and fasts.

C. Awareness that the eating pattern is abnormal and fear of not being able to stop eating voluntarily.

D. Depressed mood and self-deprecating thoughts following eating binges.

E. The bulimic episodes are not due to anorexia nervosa or any known physical disorder.

Bulimia has become an area of much concern in more affluent Western cultures,[6] but its prevalence among young Australian women remains relatively unknown. Abraham et al. recently reported that 17% of a small student sample experienced an episode of binge-eating at least once per week.[24] The aim of the present study was to estimate the prevalence of bulimia in an Australian university sample and its relationship to such variables as sex and weight using a questionnaire adapted from that used by Halmi et al.[15] The present findings are contrasted with those of Halmi and her colleagues, who surveyed students at a university in New York. Similar statistical procedures are employed in the current investigation to facilitate the comparison of data.

Method

Questionnaire

The data were obtained using a 23-item questionnaire adapted from Halmi et al.[15] The questionnaire elicited information concerning a) demographic data; b) D.S.M. III diagnostic criteria for bulimia (Table 1); c) frequency of various behaviours used to control weight and d) fluctuations in weight over a 12-month period. Subjects were also requested to define their current weight according to one of the following categories: very underweight; underweight; average; overweight; very overweight.

Subjects

The questionnaire was distributed to 678 students enrolled in undergraduate psychology courses during the Trinity Term at the University of Sydney. The statistics reported in this study reflect the responses of 303 individuals (44.7%) who completed the questionnaire.

The ages of the students ranged from 17 to 59 years with a mean age of 21.98 years and a standard deviation of 6.45 (median 19.53 years). There were 97 males (32%) and 206 females (68%). Their current weight reported in the questionnaire was converted to a percentage of standard bodyweight[25] for their reported age, sex and height (i.e. reported current weight × 100/standard bodyweight) and categorized in Table 2 along with their own definition of their current weight.

The self-defined and calculated weight categorizations were significantly correlated (Pearson r = 0.487, p < 0.001). None of the individuals who returned the questionnaire was in the objectively defined severely underweight category and only 1 respondent reported having suffered from anorexia nervosa in the past. No significant sex differences were observed in the objectively defined weight categories based upon the percentage of standard bodyweight. However, in the self-defined weight categories, females reported themselves as overweight while males reported themselves as underweight.

Table 2. Self-classification of weight and classification by percentage of standard bodyweight.

Percentage of standard bodyweight	Classification of weight	Self-classified weight category*		Category calculated by converting weight into percentage of standard bodyweight+	
		Male	Female	Male	Female
0% to 70%	very underweight	0.0%	1.0%	0.0%	0.0%
70% to 85%	underweight	23.7%	7.3%	4.2%	8.6%
85% to 110%	average	57.7%	51.7%	77.1%	69.7%
110% to 120%	overweight	15.5%	38.5%	13.5%	15.7%
> 120%	very overweight	3.1%	1.5%	5.2%	6.1%

* Item not completed in 1 case.
+ Item not completed in 9 cases.

Results

Factor Analysis

A principal-components analysis with varimax rotation produced 6 factors with eigenvalues greater than one which are presented in Table 3.

The first factor comprised the variables concerning weight, *viz.* present weight expressed as a percentage of standard bodyweight, classification of weight based upon the percentage of standard bodyweight, highest and lowest weights expressed as percentage of standard bodyweight at current height, and self-classification of weight, all of which are highly correlated although, as indicated above, self-classification of weight category is systematically biased in different directions according to sex.

The second factor represented the core symptoms of bulimia: considering oneself to be a binge-eater, short periods of time between binges, getting uncontrollable urges to eat and eat until feeling physically ill and reporting that there are times when one is afraid that one cannot stop eating voluntarily. Feeling miserable and annoyed after an eating binge also loaded on this factor but not as highly as on factor 5.

The third factor to emerge represented the clustering of variables related to dieting and purging. Whereas Halmi *et al.* found frequency of diuretic use to be unrelated to other weight-control measures,[15] in the Australian sample it was related to frequency of appetite suppressant and laxative consumption as well as self-induced vomiting. The fourth factor represented the remaining variables relating to vomiting. Unlike the New York data, in the Sydney sample other eating problems loaded with weight change over a 12-month period on the fifth factor. Abnormal eating behaviour, other than bulimia, was reported by 42 respondents (13.86% of the sample) and consisted mainly of self-deprecated behaviours such as 'eating too much junk food', although 4 subjects reported food allergies. Relatively infrequent episodes of gorging and feeling miserable and annoyed with oneself after an eating binge also loaded positively on this factor. Factor 6 represented sex differences, mainly in terms of males being taller than females, with some low loadings for females seeing themselves as overweight (while males see themselves as underweight) and as miserable and annoyed about binge-eating.

Prevalence of Bulimic Symptoms

Of the 303 persons who completed the questionnaire, 6.9% (21 subjects) acknowledged that they experienced all the major symptoms of bulimia. All 21 subjects were female (whereas Halmi *et al.*[15] found that 6 of their 46 bulimics were male).

Table 3. Principal components analysis: the six components with eigenvalues greater than one.

	Factor 1 (Weight)	Factor 2 (Bulimia)	Factor 3 (Dieting and Purging)	Factor 4 (Vomiting)	Factor 5 (Abnormal eating behaviour)	Factor 6 (Sex differences)	Communality
Present weight as percentage of standard weight	.9672*	.0386	.0162	-.0082	.0356	-.0177	.9388
Calculated weight category	.8936*	.0276	-.0415	-.0342	.0240	.0543	.8057
Highest weight at current height as percentage of standard weight	.8919*	.1609	.0928	.0284	.1303	.1021	.8582
Lowest weight at current height as percentage of standard weight	.8889*	.0472	-.0264	.0166	-.1451	-.1051	.8254
Self-classification of weight	.5979*	.2104	.1138	-.0684	.2578	.2684	.5579
Consider oneself a binge eater	.1546	.7593*	.0771	.1254	.2199	.0559	.6736
Length of time between binges	.0134	.7117*	-.1385	.1155	.4043	.1375	.7216
Uncontrollable urge to eat	.0843	.7076*	.0226	.0497	.3732	-.0268	.6507
Fear of being unable to stop eating	.1089	.6579*	.0317	.0570	.2461	.1609	.5353
Frequency of diuretic use	-.0039	.0365	.8584*	.0272	.0431	-.0059	.7409
Frequency of appetite suppressant use	.0487	-.0117	.8450*	.0964	.0851	.0462	.7352
Frequency of laxative use	.0428	.1701	.6545*	.0772	.0330	.0807	.4727
Self-induced vomiting	-.0286	.2340	.5419*	.5259	.0350	.0421	.6287
Frequency of vomiting	-.0346	.1431	.1949	.8959*	.0284	-.0237	.8637
Ever vomited after a meal	.0014	-.0888	.0200	.8948*	.0469	-.0750	.8168
Had a binge episode	.0615	.1681	.0899	-.0547	.7213*	-.0971	.5727
Feel miserable and annoyed after a binge	.2563	.3933	.0860	.0006	.5281*	.2754	.5825
Any other type of eating problem	-.1956	.0163	.0228	.0200	.5058*	.1617	.3214
Amount of weight change during the past year	.1984	.1558	.0393	.1313	.4215*	-.0227	.2606
Height	-.1595	.0425	-.0067	.0201	.0270	-.8310*	.7189
Sex (+ = female)	-.0566	.1152	.0258	-.0582	.1267	.8292*	.7242
Accounted variance	18.58%	11.37%	10.86%	9.34%	8.46%	7.87%	66.48%

*Highest raw loading

Table 4. Prevalence of symptoms of bulimia and vomiting in male and female university students.

Questions relating to binge-eating and vomiting	Affirmative responses (Male and female)	Affirmative responses by sex		Chi square	P (df = 1)
		Male	Female		
A. Binge-eating					
Uncontrollable urge to eat	24.1%	17.7%	27.1%	2.648	n.s.
Episode of an eating binge	60.7%	52.6%	64.6%	3.486	n.s.
Cannot voluntarily stop eating	18.5%	9.4%	22.8%	6.967	0.0083
Feeling miserable and annoyed	43.8%	23.4%	53.2%	21.984	<0.00005
Consider self a binge-eater	16.5%	8.2%	20.4%	6.201	0.0128
B. Vomiting					
Ever vomited after eating	28.7%	35.4%	25.5%	2.651	n.s.
Self-induced vomiting	4.0%	3.1%	4.4%	0.047	n.s.

There was a female preponderance for the following bulimia variables: feeling miserable and annoyed with oneself after an eating binge, being afraid at times that one cannot stop eating voluntarily and considering oneself a binge-eater (see Table 4).

The mean number of days between episodes of binge-eating was 39 days (standard deviation 59.6 days) for the 109 subjects who reported bingeing. The range was 1 to 365 days (median 20.4 days, mode 30 days). The number of days between episodes of binge-eating correlated significantly with considering oneself a binge-eater (-0.335, p.< 0.001), getting uncontrollable urges to eat and eat until one feels physically ill (-0.264, p = 0.006) and being afraid at times that one cannot stop eating voluntarily (-0.222, p = 0.021) but not with self-classification of weight. The number of days between eating binges decreases if the subjects consider themselves to be binge-eaters, get uncontrollable urges to eat or fear that they cannot stop eating.

There was a significant correlation between the weight variables and the symptoms of bulimia, the average correlation being 0.226 (p < 0.01). Self-categorisation of weight was different for those reporting bulimic symptoms compared with those who did not (p < 0.001), with those reporting bulimic symptoms seeing themselves as overweight in keeping with the preponderance of females shown in Table 4 (males, in general, report themselves as underweight). However, those individuals who reported symptoms of bulimia did tend to have a history of higher weight (present, highest and lowest weights as percentages of standard weight for present height) than those who did not experience bulimic symptoms.

Frequency of Vomiting and of Medication Use

Vomiting on at least one occasion after eating was reported by 87 people (28.7%) while 4% of the sample indicated that they had induced vomiting (Table 4). However, only 1.2% (1 person, a female) did so one or more times a day. More males acknowledged vomiting after eating than their female counterparts but this may be associated with higher consumption of alcohol in males. There was no significant relationship between self-induced vomiting and the weight variables, neither self-reported weight category nor present weight as a percentage of standard bodyweight is related to self-induced vomiting. Thus self-induced vomiting has a low incidence, there is no significant sex bias and no relationship between self-induced vomiting and weight history. However, there was a significant correlation ($p = 0.001$) between frequency of vomiting and the frequency of use of appetite suppressants (used by 4.6% of the sample), diuretics (used by 3.6%) and laxatives (used by 7.6%). Other forms of weight control included exercise which was reportedly taken regularly by 5% of the sample, while 4.6% dieted, 2.3% used various forms of diet supplements such as vitamin tablets and 1.4% belonged to a weight control group (Table 5).

Of the persons who reported self-induced vomiting, 41.7% (5 persons) also experienced all the major symptoms of bulimia.

Discussion

It has recently been suggested that the number of bulimic patients seeking treatment may only '... represent the tip of the iceberg of a much more widespread morbidity within the general population'.[26] However, there have been relatively

Table 5. Frequency of vomiting and of the use of appetite suppressants, laxatives and diuretics in the university sample.

	Use of			
	appetite suppressants	laxatives	diuretics	vomiting
Never	95.4%	92.4%	96.4%	70.3%
Less than one per month	1.7%	4.3%	1.0%	23.4%
1 to 3 times a week	0.7%	1.0%	0.0%	0.0%
1 or more times a week	1.7%	1.3%	1.0%	1.3%
Not reported	0.7%	1.0%	1.7%	5.0%

few reports in the recent literature concerning the epidemiology of bulimia and the findings reported are inconsistent.

The findings of the present investigation indicate a lower incidence of bulimia, at least in Australia, than previously suggested by some authors,[15,23,24] and are more consistent with the results reported by Pyle et al.[27] who found that 4% of the student population of a state university in the American midwest met the DSM III diagnosis of bulimia. The present results also agree with those of Stangler and Printz who reported that 3.8% of 500 consecutive students (89.5% female, 10.5% male) assessed and treated at a university health clinic met the relevant criteria for a diagnosis of bulimia to be made.[21]

There appears to be a marked variation in the prevalence of bulimia in student populations ranging from a conservative 3.8%[21] to 20% reported by Wooley and Wooley.[23] The degree of variation probably reflects the heterogeneity of student populations investigated (those attending summer school or health clinics), the percentage of students participating in research projects of this nature, different interpretations of core symptoms[28] and the validity of their responses. It is generally accepted that patients with bulimia are secretive concerning their gorging and/or purgative behaviour[11] and surveys completed may be an underestimation of the actual incidence of this disorder. In addition, only 44.7% of the students surveyed in the present investigation completed the questionnaire and this may also have contributed towards the lower incidence of bulimia.

With the exception of the prevalence of bulimia, the results of the present investigation confirm most of the findings reported by Halmi et al.[15] in their survey of students at a campus of the State University of New York: a) individuals reporting symptoms of bulimia had a history of being overweight, compared with their standard bodyweight, or were over-represented among those currently weighing 110% or more of standard weight; b) there was a low incidence of self-induced vomiting, no definite sex bias and no significant relationship between self-induced vomiting and weight variables; c) a positive correlation between self-induced vomiting and laxative abuse; d) females saw themselves as being overweight whilst males considered themselves underweight. Halmi et al.[15] found that the use of diuretics was not significantly related to either bingeing or vomiting. However, we found an association between the use of diuretics, appetite suppressants and purgatives.

The present study thus provides further support for the notion that although self-induced vomiting may accompany symptoms of bulimia, it is not a necessary criterion for the diagnosis of the disorder.[11,15] Abraham and Beumont described the behaviour and symptoms of 32 patients who presented at an eating disorders clinic complaining of episodes of voracious overeating which they felt was out of their control.[11] They were able to divide them into 'vomiters' and 'non-vomiters'. The vomiters tended to have a longer duration of illness but they did not have significantly different permorbid weights from the non-vomiters. This is consistent with the present results where there was no significant correlation between self-induced vomiting and weight variables. However, this does not appear to hold true for patients with anorexia nervosa where the 'vomiters and purgers' had significantly different weight histories from the 'non-vomiters'.[12,29] The 'vomiters and purgers' tended to be overweight premorbidly. It is interesting to note that 5% of the sample reported exercising as a means of weight control compared with the 4.6% who dieted. Jogging is currently viewed as a healthy and highly desirable behaviour[30] and it is therefore not surprising that compulsive overexercising in patients with anorexia nervosa is becoming more prevalent.[31]

Recent research has focused upon developing more effective techniques to manage the increasing number of individuals presenting for treatment, [32-36] but the long-term outcome of bulimia remains controversial.

References

1. Schwarz, D.M.; Thompson, M.G. and Johnson, C.L.: Anorexia nervosa and bulimia: the socio-cultural context. *International Journal of Eating Disorders* 1 (3): 20-36 (1982).
2. Casper, R.C.: On the emergence of bulimia nervosa as a syndrome: a historical review. *International Journal of Eating Disorders* 2 (3): 3-16 (1983).
3. Garner, D.M. and Garfinkel, P.E.: Sociocultural factors in anorexia nervosa. *Lancet* (Sept): 674 (1978).
4. Garner, D.M.; Garfinkel, P.E.; Schwartz, D. and Thompson, M.: The cultural expectations of thinness in women. *Psychological Reports* 47: 483-91 (1983).
5. Johnson, C.L.; Stuckey, M.K.; Lewis, L.D. and Schwartz, D.M.: Bulimia: a descriptive survey of 316 cases. *International Journal of Eating Disorders* 2 (1): 3-16 (1982).
6. Kalucy, R.S.: Eating disorders in young women. *Medical Journal of Australia* 2: 205-6 (1983).
7. Touyz, S.W.; Beumont, P.J.V.; Collins, J.K.; McCabe, M. and Jupp, J.: Body shape perception and disturbance in anorexia nervosa. *British Journal of Psychiatry* 144: 167-71 (1984).
8. American Psychiatric Association: *Diagnostic and Statistical Manual of Mental Disorders* 3rd (A.P.A., Washington, D.C. 1979)
9. Stunkard, A.J.: Eating patterns and obesity. *Psychiatric Quarterly*. 33: 284-95 (1959).
10. Wermuth, B.H.; Davis, K.L.; Hollister, L.E. and Stunkard, A.J.: Phenytoin treatment of the binge eating syndrome. *American Journal of Psychiatry* 134: 1249-53 (1977).
11. Abraham, S.F. and Beumont, P.J.V.: How patients describe bulimia or binge eating. *Psychological Medicine* 12: 625-35 (1982).
12. Beumont, P.J.V.; George, G.C.W. and Smart, D.E.: 'Dieters' and 'vomiters and purgers' in anorexia nervosa. *Psychological Medicine*, 6: 617-22 (1976).
13. Casper, R.C.; Eckert, E.D.; Halmi, K.A.; Goldberg, S.C. and Davis, J.M.: The incidence and clinical significance of bulimia in patients with anorexia nervosa. *Archives of General Psychiatry* 37: 1030-5 (1980).
14. Garfinkel, P.E.; Moldofsky, H. and Garner, D.M.: The heterogeneity of anorexia nervosa. *Archives of General Psychiatry* 37: 1036-40 (1980).
15. Halmi, K.A.; Falk, J.R. and Schwartz, E.: Binge-eating and vomiting: a survey of a college population. *Psychological Medicine* 11: 697-706 (1981).

16. Hawkins, R.C. and Clement, P.F.: Development and construct validation of a self report measure of binge-eating tendencies. *Addictive Behaviours* 5: 219-26 (1980).

17. Holmgren, S.; Humble, K.; Norking, C.; Roos, B.; Rosmark, B. and Sohlberg, S.: The anorectic bulimic conflict. *International Journal of Eating Disorders* 2: (2) 3-14 (1983).

18. Lacey, J.H.: The bulimic syndrome at normal body weight: reflections on pathogenesis and clinical features. *International Journal of Eating Disorders* 2 (1): 59-66 (1982).

19. Pyle, R.L.; Mitchell, J.E.: and Eckert, E.D.: Bulimia: a report of 34 cases. *Journal of Clinical Psychiatry* 42 (2): 10-64 (1981).

20. Russell, G.: Bulimia nervosa: an ominous variant of anorexia nervosa. *Psychological Medicine* 9: 429-48 (1979).

21. Stangler, R.S. and Printz, A.M.: D.S.M. III: psychiatric diagnosis in a university population. *American Journal of Psychiatry* 137: 937-40 (1980).

22. Thompson, M. and Schwartz, D.: Life adjustment of women with anorexia nervosa and anorexic-like behavior. *International Journal of Eating Disorders*, 2 (1): 47-60 (1981).

23. Wooley, O.W. and Wooley, S.: The Beverly Hills Eating Disorders: the mass marketing of anorexia nervosa. *International Journal of Eating Disorders* 1 (3): 57-69 (1982).

24. Abraham, S.F.; Mira, H.; Beumont, P.J.V.; Sowerbutts, T.D. and Llewellyn-Jones, D.: Eating behaviours among young women. *Medical Journal of Australia* 2: 225-8 (1983).

25. Society of Actuaries. *Build and Blood Pressure Study*. Vol. 1. (Society of Actuaries, Chicago 1959).

26. Crisp, A.H.: Anorexia nervosa at normal body weight: the abnormal normal weight control syndrome. *International Journal of Psychiatry in Medicine* 11: 203-33 (1982).

27. Pyle, R.L.; Mitchell, J.E.; Eckert, E.C.; Halvorson, P.A.; Neuman, P.A. and Goff, G.M.: The incidence of bulimia in freshmen college students. *International Journal of Eating Disorders* 2 (3): 75-86 (1983).

28. Fairburn, C.G. and Cooper, D.J.: The epidemiology of bulimia nervosa. *International Journal of Eating Disorders* 2: (4) 61-7 (1983).

29. Beumont, P.J.V.: Further categorization of patients with anorexia nervosa. *Australian and New Zealand Journal of Psychiatry*, 11: 223-6 (1977).

30. Yates, A.; Leehey, K. and Shisslak, C.M.: Running – an analogue of anorexia? *New England Journal of Medicine* 308: 251-5 (1983).

31. Beumont, P.J.V.; Touyz, S.W. and Hook, S.: Excessive exercise in anorexia nervosa. *Proceedings of the International Conference on Anorexia Nervosa and Related Disorders*, Swansea 1984.

32. Cinciripini, P.M.; Kornblith, S.J.; Turner, S.M. and Hersen, M.: A behavioural programme for the management of anorexia nervosa and bulimia. *Journal of Nervous and Mental Disease* 171: 186-9 (1983).

33. Fairburn, C.G.: The place of a cognitive behavioral approach in the management of bulimia; in Barby, Garfinkel, Garner and Coscina (Eds) *Anorexia Nervosa: Recent Developments in Research*, (Alan Liss, New York 1983).

34. Johnson, C.; Connors, M. and Stuckey, M.: Short-term group treatment of bulimia. *International Journal of Eating Disorders* 2 (4): 199-208 (1983).

35. Lacey, J.H.: Bulimia nervosa, binge eating and psychogenic vomiting: a controlled treatment study and long term outcome. *British Medical Journal* 286: 1609-13 (1983).

36. Long, C.G. and Cordle, C.J.: Psychological treatment of binge eating and self-induced vomiting. *British Journal of Medical Psychology* 55: 139-45 (1982).

Chapter VII

Bulimia: Therapy at a Distance

Introduction

There has been an increase in the number of reports of binge eating among non-patient populations, [1-6] and of studies to determine the prevalence of bulimia among non-patients. [7-11] Although these reports elucidate the discrepancies between the frequency of binge eating and the number who seek medical treatment for it, there are few, if any, attempts to delineate the characteristics of those who seek such treatment from those who do not.

Perhaps, not surprisingly, the early identification of bulimia as an independent syndrome focused upon the binge eating among the obese in hospital, [12,13] and among patients with anorexia nervosa, [14-19] where there have been attempts to identify a subgroup of these patients who have bulimic symptoms. [17, 20-22] Despite the numerous assertions that bulimia has become widespread, [1-3, 5,16, 23-32] and that those who present for treatment represent 'only the tip of the iceberg', [27] an alternative viewpoint is that although growing evidence supports a sociocultural interpretation, it may have led to the overzealous detection by clinicians and the over-identification of the psychiatric condition among those without serious psychopathology. [33,34]

The validity of claims that bulimia is a distinct psychiatric syndrome remains obscure because every school child knows that bingeing was and still is widespread. The inevitable bias that results from simple descriptions of selected groups without comparing them directly with non-patients further obscures the features that might make such behaviour pathological. Epidemiologists have long pointed out that studies of clinical conditions in hospital patients are liable to distortion because of selection factors unrelated to the illnesses themselves. Such a selection process begins at the point of entry into primary care, and there is a widespread belief that illness is not the only factor that determines whether people consult professionals for treatment.

Although there is still a paucity of reports that describe the treatment of bulimia, one of the most firmly established facts from the outcome literature is that there are large individual differences in responsiveness to treatment. Some bulimics improve markedly, others show some improvement, and still others seem to be unchanged or worse after treatment. Such a discrepancy in response might not be surprising if it is the case that motivation to seek or to participate in treatment is also highly discrepant. It is well known, of course, that a large proportion of individuals with anorexia nervosa do not want, nor do they see the reason for, treatment. It would obviously be valuable if clinicians could determine which individuals would respond to treatment, or better, to specific treatments. Those who have not been, or do not wish to be, treated can provide important information about the nature and the motivation of those who do seek help for bulimia. Granted that there is a great variability among subjects in their responsivity to treatment, valuable insights into the nature and treatment of bulimia might be gained from an examination of subject variables, or characteristics that are predictive of compliance within treatment, and of success or failure in programmes for bulimia.

Such descriptions might also tell us why bulimia poses difficulties for clinicians and is often thought to be resistant to treatment. The crucial importance of understanding the apparently intractible nature of bulimia in some individuals is well recognized. An important omission in the bulimia literature is research that investigates the process and primary determinants of relapse.

While it might seem reasonable to assume that the severity of any symptom determines whether bulimics ask for help, other factors that might influence that decision include the reactions of others, the distress that results from bingeing, its resistance to self-directed change, and a search for insight into what is involved. Whatever their reasons, the fact that so many 'bulimics' do not appear to seek help compels us to investigate the distinctions between 'bulimic' patients and non-patients, in order to clarify how, if at all, bingers who seek help differ from those who engage in the same behaviour but who do not wish to be 'treated' for it.

It could be, as Lucas [30] has suggested, that the vast majority of affected individuals are satisfactorily adjusted and lead apparently normal lives, although they purposely control their weight by vomiting or purging. On the other hand these people could represent an undetected source of psychiatric morbidity. [35] Nevertheless, some researchers have noted that, despite the severity of the bingeing and purging behaviour, a large proportion of individuals does not seek professional help. So Fairburn and Cooper reported that although 80% of their community-based sample considered they had an eating problem only 2.5% were receiving treatment, and Johnson *et al.* [8] found 56% of their respondents had not sought professional help.

The present study, part of an ongoing investigation into the function, usefulness and optimal characteristics of minimal therapist contact and self-help for bulimia (an analysis and a description of the outcome of this programme, based on procedures found to be effective in a clinical setting, is in press)[36] was designed to identify the characteristics of women who requested detailed information about bulimia and those who enquired but declined to receive the material. Further comparisons are possible between those who have stayed in this programme and those who have dropped out at an earlier stage. The second component of the present report, therefore, attempts to identify determinants of 'non-compliance' among women who agreed initially to participate in a self-help programme for bulimia.

Method

The source of these data is in replies to a request in *Dolly* magazine in January 1983, following an interview that they reported, to write in for information about bulimia. In response to that invitation letters were received from over 150 women, all of whom were sent a questionnaire concerning their eating, weight-related behaviour and attitudes and a Body Cathexis and Self Cathexis measure.[37] These were to be returned in a pre-paid envelope. They were asked if they would like to participate in a mailing programme designed to provide information about how to overcome their bulimia. Responses to the questionnaires from the first 100 respondents who were not at that time receiving any treatment for their bulimia form the data for this chapter.

Results

The results will be presented in 3 sections. The first section describes the salient characteristics of the total sample, in comparison with comparable results from Fairburn's [35] analysis of the information he gathered in a similar way in Britain. The other sections compare the responses of those who agreed to participate in the programme with those who did not, and the responses of those who continued in the programme with those who began but dropped out from it. Finally these Australian results will be compared with Abraham and Beumont's [38] data (the only detailed account of bulimia in Australia that has been published so far) from 30 of their female bulimic patients.

All of the letters were from women, of whom 15% were married, 4% divorced or separated and 81% single. Their ages ranged from 15 to 42 with a mean of 22.1 years.

Weight characteristics

Seventy-five per cent of these women reported a current weight that fell between 85% and 115% of their standard body weight as can be seen from Table 1, with the mean weight of the series being 56.58kg. A notable feature of these results is the differences in these current and desired weights from those in Fairburn's sample of 449 British women. Of the women in his study, 11% reported a desired weight that was less than 75% of their standard body weight, yet none of the women in the present study wished to weigh less than 75% of their standard weight. While 16% of those in this study had a desired weight between 75% and 85% of their standard weight, Fairburn reported that this was the case for 52% in his. None of the British women said they wished to weigh more than their standard weight, yet 26% of the women in this series reported a desired weight between 100% and 115% of their standard weight. This discrepancy is consistent with other differences in the percentages whose current weights were above 115% (16% in this series and 5.5% in Fairburn's) and between 100% and 115% (42% in this study and 29.2% in Fairburn's). Although the differences in minimum

Table 1. Distribution of women in the present series (n=100) and in that of Fairburn (n=499)[35] in different weight groups according to their present and desired weights, and their minimum and maximum weights since menarche.

Weight category (% of SBW)*	Per cent of women							
	Present weight		Weight since menarche				Desired weight	
	H[†]	F[‡]	Highest		Lowest		H	F
			H	F	H	F		
75	1%	1%	0 %	0.2%	11%	12.4%	0%	11.2%
75 to 85	8%	10.5%	0%	0%	29%	30.6%	16%	52.0%
86 to 100	33%	54%	8%	9.7%	44%	50.3%	58%	36.9%
101 to 115	42%	29.2%	34%	44.8%	13%	6.4%	26%	0%
115	16%	5.5%	58%	45.2%	3%	0.2%	0%	0%

* Per cent of standard weight for age and height.
† The present series.
‡ Figures taken directly from Fairburn's series. [35]

Table 2. Direct comparison of Fairburn's (1982) British magazine results [35] with the Australian Dolly series.

	Fairburn n=499	Huon n=100
Mean age (years)		
Present age	23.8	22.1
Onset of binge eating	18.4	17.2
Duration	5.2	4.5
Onset of vomiting	19.2	18.2
Frequency of binge eating (%)		
Daily	27.2%	25.0%
Weekly	32.6%	68.0%
Frequency of vomiting (%)		
Daily	56.1%	52.0%
Weekly	17.5%	17.0%
Purgation (%)	18.8%	29.0%
Loss of control over eating (%)	63.0%	79.0%
Secrecy about vomiting (%)	38.7%	33.0%
Previous anorexia nervosa* (%)	43.0%	40.0%

* Women who reported a lowest weight of less than 85% of their standard body weight and accompanying amenorrhoea.

and maximum weights are not pronounced there is a trend for the Australian women to be heavier, and so more likely to be overweight. That could reflect differences in living standards here and in Britain, or it could result from differences in the way the 2 invitations were worded. Fairburn, who did not specify which magazine he used, specifically asked those who used self-induced vomiting as a means of weight control to write to him while the Dolly interview asked about bulimia.

The mean current age, as well as the mean age at the onset of bingeing and at the onset of vomiting were somewhat younger in this study (Table 2). Although the proportion of women who reported at least a daily binge in each sample is similar (27.2% in Fairburn's study and 25.0% in this study), 68% of the present series were bingeing at least weekly compared with only 32.6% of the British women. The reported frequency of vomiting (56% in Fairburn's study and 52% in the present study) shows little difference, although 18.8% of women in Fairburn's series and 29% of these women said they use purgatives.

An important question when one is looking at bulimia, which may also occur 'normally', is what marks off those who want to change, from those who don't. To identify what might characterize those 2 groups the sample was divided into those who did *not* actually enter the programme (Group 1; N=24) and those who did (Group 2; N=76).

As is shown in Table 3, there are significant mean differences between groups 1 and 2 in their maximum and minimum weights as well as in their weights prior to the onset of bingeing. The women who decided to participate had higher weights in each of those categories, although they did not differ significantly in their current, standard, and desired weights.

Furthermore, the women who did not participate in the programme said they began dieting, bingeing and vomiting earlier than did the others, as can be seen in Table 4.

Table 3. Mean values of the characteristics of those who wrote in following the Dolly interview.

	Group 1* n=24	Group 2† n=76	2a‡ n=19	2b§ n=50‖
Current height (m)	1.62	1.60	1.61	1.60
Current weight (kg)	53.73	56.93++	54.14	57.96 $p < 0.05$
Standard weight (kg)	54.82	55.11	53.74	54.68
Maximum weight (kg)	60.55	67.58 $p < 0.01$	63.82	68.43 $p < 0.05$
Minimum weight (kg)	44.50	51.32 $p < 0.01$	46.35	51.76 $p < 0.01$
Weight prior to onset of bingeing (kg)	56.70	60.01 $p < 0.01$	58.87	61.50 $p < 0.005$
Desired weight (kg)	48.19	52.12	49.77	52.61

* Declined.
† Accepted the programme.
‡ Withdrew after second mailing.
§ Have stayed in the programme.
‖ 7 women are late in their participation.
++ The mean current weight of Abraham and Beumont's [37] 30 female patients was 55.2kg.

Table 4. Mean ages of the groups in the present series compared with patients in Abraham and Beumont's report.[37]

	Group 1 n=24	Group 2 n=76	2a n=19	2b n=50	Patients n=30
Present age	20.5	22.6	20.6	23.3	24.2
Age when began dieting	14.29	15.58 $p < 0.01$	15.1	16.3 $p < 0.05$	–
Age at onset of bingeing	16.4	17.4 $p < 0.05$	16.3	17.2 $p < 0.01$	17.0
Age at onset of vomiting	16.6	18.7 $p < 0.001$	18.5	18.9	–

Table 5. Bingeing behaviour.

	Per cent of women				
	Group 1 n=24	Group 2 n=76	2a n=19	2b n=50	Patients n=30
Frequency of bingeing					
At least daily	70.5%	68.4%	47.4%	58.4%	'variable'
At least weekly	29.5%	25.0%	31.6%	22.9%	from hours
At least monthly	0%	6.6%	21.0%	18.7%	to weeks
Average length of binge					
≤ 1 hour	70.8%	50.0%	51.6%	50.0%	'variable' from 15
> 1 hour	29.2%	50.0% p < 0.05	48.4%	50.0%	mins to 3 weeks
Control during binge					
Some control if choose	26.1%	17.1%	36.8%	12.0%	'depersonalization'
Completely out of control	73.9%	82.9%	63.2%	88. 0% p < 0.02	75.0%
Binges planned					
Mostly, always	78.2%	61.8%	52.6%	66.0%	75.0%
Rarely, never	21.8%	38.2% p < 0.05	47.4%	34.0%	
Do you disguise your bingeing?					
Yes	75.0%	93.3%	94.7%	91.8%	23.3%
No	25.0%	6.7% p < 0.05	5.3%	8.2%	
Precipitants					
Specific foods					
Rarely, never	58.3%	65.4%	21.1%	50.0%	
Mostly, always	41.7%	34.6%	78.9%	50.0 % p < 0.05	78.0%
Arguments					
With family	29.4%	43.1%	50.0%	70.6%	'less frequent than
With others	70.6%	66.9%	50.0%	29.4 % p < 0.05	22.0%'
Anxious during binge					
Rarely, never	37.5%	36.0%	52.6%	24.6%	72.0%
Mostly, always	62.5%	64.0%	47.4%	75.5 % p < 0.05	

An examination of the bingeing behaviour in groups 1 and 2 (Table 5) reveals significant differences in the average length of a binge-eating episode, in the ability or desire to disguise the behaviour, and in whether the binges were planned or not. The frequency of the binges, the reported anxiety and lack of control during a binge, and the factors that were said to precipitate an episode of bingeing were all very similar.

There was no significant difference in the frequency of self-induced vomiting, although 47.4% of group 1 compared with 26.0% of group 2 use purgatives when bingeing, and a significantly larger number in group 1 said they had told someone about their vomiting or purging.

Those who entered the programme were further divided into those who dropped out (Group 2a; N=19) and those who have remained in the programme (Group 2b; N=50). It is important to explain the apparent discrepancies in numbers who continued to participate. The programme consisted of 7 monthly components which combined information, structured exploration and task-oriented suggestions for change in attitudes and behaviours relating to food, the body and self concepts. In addition, a brief questionnaire for the progressive monitoring of changes and of reactions to the programme was to be returned each month. Seven women in the programme have been removed from the analysis at this stage. For reasons of travel, illness or study they are somewhat out of phase, despite their desire to remain in the programme, and it was believed to be appropriate not to include them as 'in' or 'out' since their 'status' is somewhat ambiguous.

Another very interesting finding concerns the reasons for dropping out. The initial phase of this programme requires that participants systematically monitor their bingeing. Reactions to that task generally assume an important focus for discussion in the early stages of treatment for bulimia in the clinical setting. Acknowledging the significance of this, the early material mailed to the participants encouraged them to consider their reactions to that task. All 19 women who dropped out from the programme did so after the second mailing, and when asked in a follow-up questionnaire about the reasons for their dropping out, all of them noted their resistance to, difficulty with and resentment about being expected to record their bingeing. Many commented that it is easier to 'pretend it is not happening,' or that once it is examined carefully they feared that they would have to 'give it up'. Of those who did offer these comments 7 women asked if they could have another opportunity to participate in the programme. Resistance to filling out bingeing sheets has also been noted by Johnson et al.[39], and of course the reactivity of self-monitoring has been a topic of major interest in the area of smoking research. [40]

It can be seen from Table 3 that those women who have continued in the programme show higher mean current, maximum and minimum weights and higher mean weight prior to the onset of bingeing than those who dropped out.

In addition, although there is no significant difference in their current age, or in their age at the onset of vomiting, those women who have dropped out began dieting and bingeing at a significantly younger age (Table 4).

There are again no significant differences in the frequency or the length of bingeing episodes, yet the stated precipitants of a binge, and the anxiety experienced during bingeing both showed significant differences between the drop-out and the continuing groups. Those who dropped out said more frequently that eating specific foods triggered a binge, while those who have stayed in said that arguments with members of their family precipitated bingeing. These findings bear on those of Norman and Herzog, [41] whose bulimic patients also had significantly elevated scores on 'troubled family relations'. Whereas 47.4% of those who have dropped out experienced anxiety during bingeing, 75.5% of those who are still in the programme said that they felt anxious. Although the questionnaire asked about anxiety, depression, lack of self worth before, during and after bingeing, anxiety during the binge was the only item that revealed significant differences in any of these comparisons.

There were, similarly, no significant differences in the frequency of self-induced vomiting or in the use of purgatives between these 2 groups.

In order to further define what, if any, are the similarities and differences between these groups of women in the study and a sample of bulimic patients, data from the 30 women in Abraham and Beumont's [38] study were examined. Where comparable data are available they have been included in Table 6. The mean weight of their patients when they presented was 55.2kg, which lies between those in the present series who dropped out and those who remained. Although the mean age of the patients at presentation is slightly older, their age at the onset of bingeing was 17 years, which is the same as those who have stayed in the programme.

It is not possible to directly compare the frequency and length of the binge-eating episodes between these patients and those in the present series, since Abraham and Beumont emphasize the variability in the length of, and the time between, binges and note that a long history of bingeing seemed to be associated with describing the binges as lasting for days or for weeks. Perhaps the most notable differences are in the mood disturbances that were reported by their patients, all of whom said they usually felt anxious and tense *before* a binge, while 75% reported feelings of depersonalization. These figures compare with the 47% in the present study who said they always felt anxious before bingeing, and

Table 6. Vomiting and purging behaviour.

	Per cent of women				
	Group 1 n=24	Group 2 n=76	2a n=19	2b n=50	Patients n=30
Induce vomiting					
Mostly, always	40.6%	44.7%	42.1%	46.0%	
Rarely, never	59.4%	55.3%	57.9	54.0%	53.0%
Purgation					
Rarely, never	52.6%	74.0%	79.1%	68.4%	
Mostly, always	47.4%	26.0% p < 0.05	20.9%	31.6%	73.0%
Anyone know about your purging?					
Yes	86.4%	55.9%	43.8%	60.0%	
No	13.6%	44.1% p < 0.01	56.2%	40.0%	n.a.

with the 88% of those who have remained in the programme who said they feel totally out of control during a binge. This is the closest to a direct comparison with the feelings of depersonalization noted by Abraham and Beumont. Since only 23% of their patients, but 91% of these women say they disguise or perhaps conceal their behaviour, it might be that the disclosure of their symptoms, including their mood fluctuations, determines the patients' ability or desire to disguise their behaviour; this cannot of course be decided from these data. However, 70% of the patients reported thoughts of suicide after bingeing, and Abraham and Beumont note that most of their patients had come under medical care because of their abnormal body weight or a suicide attempt.

Discussion

This study is a step towards understanding the way those who seek some form of treatment for bulimia differ from those who are aware of their bingeing but do not look for help with it, despite the fact that there may be some biases in these data, because 14 of the 150 who wrote to me initially did not reply again (and of course an unknown number of bingers did not write at all).

These results suggest that major factors influencing help-seeking relate more to the distress with bingeing and purging and perhaps to the absence of any person who knows about the problem than simply to the frequency with which it occurs.

Although there were some differences in the extent of this bingeing between the groups, and between Beumont's patients and these non-patients, there was little difference in their vomiting and a significantly greater use of purgatives by the patients. Furthermore, the tension and anxiety that is associated with the patients' bingeing, and the relief of dysphoric moods following a binge might point to distress as one significant variable that differentiates bulimic patients from non-patients. Despite Abraham and Beumont's claim that an ability to induce vomiting is a major influence determining the clinical form of bulimia, the present results do not support the generality of that conclusion, since there is little difference in the frequency of self-induced vomiting among any of the groups. Russell [16] has, however, included self-induced vomiting or purging as one of his 3 diagnostic criteria for bulimia nervosa which is his preferred term for what the Americans call 'bulimia'. But it might be more constructive to distinguish simple bulimia, characterized by episodes of gross over-eating, from bulimia nervosa which requires subsequent vomiting or purging. Although Abraham and Beumont have suggested that distress surrounds whether a binger is able to vomit, it is possible that this and the distress associated with bingeing itself, and about what happens (or does not happen) then, could compound into a decision to seek treatment, or at least a wish to tell someone.

This programme of psychological treatment at a distance involves giving information and encouraging cooperation by requiring individuals to monitor and report their progress. It has been shown that the disorder may have been more, or at least equally, severe in those who did not enter the programme but that those who have stayed in may have done so because of the distress that their bingeing causes them.

References

1. Ondercin, P.A.: Compulsive eating in college women. *Journal of College Student Personnel* 20: 153-7 (1979).
2. Wardle, J.: Dietary restraint and binge eating. *Behavioural Analysis and Modification* 4: 201-9 (1980).
3. Hawkins, R.C. and Clement, P.F.: Development and construct validation of a self-report measure of binge eating tendencies. *Addictive Behaviour* 5: 219-26 (1980).
4. Halmi, K.A., Falk, J.R. and Schwartz, E.: Binge-eating and vomiting: a survey of a college population. *Psychological Medicine* 11: 697-706 (1981).
5. Edelman, B.: Binge eating in normal weight and over weight individuals. *Psychological Reports* 49: 739-46 (1981).
6. Abraham, S.F., Mira, M., Beumont, P.J.V., Sowerbutts, T.D. and Llewellyn-Jones, D.: Eating behaviour among young women. *Medical Journal of Australia* 2: 225-8 (1983).
7. Collins, M., Kreisberg, J., Pertschuk, M. and Fager, S.: Bulimia in college women. *Journal of Adolescent Health Care* 3: 144 (1982).
8. Johnson, C.L., Stuckey, M.K., Lewis, L.D. and Schwartz, D.M.: Bulimia: a descriptive survey of 316 cases. *International Journal of Eating Disorders* 2: 3-16 (1982).
9. Pyle, R.L., Mitchell, J.E., Eckert, E.E., Halvorson, P.A., Neuman, P.A. and Goff, G.M.: The incidence of bulimia in freshman college students. *International Journal of Eating Disorders* 2: 75-86 (1983).
10. Lucas, A.R., Beard, C.M., Kranz, J.S. and Kurland, L.T.: Epidemiology of anorexia nervosa and bulimia. *International Journal of Eating Disorders* 2: 85-90 (1983).
11. Fairburn, C. and Cooper, P.J.: The epidemiology of bulimia nervosa. *International Journal of Eating Disorders* 2: 61-7 (1983).
12. Stunkard, A.J.: Eating patterns and obesity. *Psychiatric Quarterly* 33: 284-92 (1959).
13. Hawkins, R.C.: Meal/snack frequencies of college students: a normative study. *Behavioural Psychotherapy* 7: 85-90 (1979).
14. Bliss, E.L. and Branch, C.H.H.: *Anorexia nervosa. Its history, psychology and biology.* Paul Hoeber Inc., New York 1960).
15. Guiora, A.Z.: Dysorexia: a psychopathological study of anorexia nervosa and bulimia. *American Journal of Psychiatry* 124: 391-3 (1967).
16. Russell, G.: Bulimia nervosa: an ominous variant of anorexia nervosa. *Psychological Medicine* 9: 429-48 (1979).
17. Casper, R.C., Halmi, K.A., Goldberg, S.C., Eckert, E. and Davis, J.M.: Anorexia nervosa and bulimia. *Archives of General Psychiatry* 39: 487-9 (1982).
18. Lowenkopf, E.L.: Anorexia nervosa: Some nosological considerations. *Comprehensive Psychiatry* 23: 233-40 (1982).
19. Strober, M., Salkin, B., Burroughs, J. and Morrell, W.: Validity of the bulimia-restricter distinction in anorexia nervosa. Parental personality characteristics and family psychiatric morbidity. *Journal of Nervous and Mental Disease* 170: 345-51 (1982).

20. Kalucy, R.S., Crisp, A.H., Lacey, J.H. and Harding, B.: Prevalence and prognosis in anorexia nervosa. *Australian and New Zealand Journal of Psychiatry* 11: 251-7 (1977).

21. Halmi, K.A., Casper, R.C., Eckert, E.D., Goldberg, S.C. and Davis, J.M.: Unique features associated with age of onset of anorexia nervosa. *Psychiatry Research* 1: 209-15 (1979).

22. Garfinkel, P.E., Moldofsky, H. and Garner, D.M.: The heterogeneicity of anorexia nervosa. Bulimia as a distinct subgroup. *Archives of General Psychiatry* 37: 1036-40 (1980).

23. Boskind-Lodahl, M.: Cinderella's stepsisters: A feminist perspective on anorexia nervosa and bulimia. *Signs* 2: 342-56 (1976).

24. Nogami, Y. and Yabana, F.: On kibarashi-gui (binge eating). *Folia Psychiatrica et Neurologica Japonica* 31: 159-66 (1977).

25. Fairburn, C.: Self-induced vomiting. *Journal of Psychosomatic Research* 24: 193-7 (1980).

26. Allerdissen, R., Florin, I. and Rost, W.: Psychological characteristics of women with bulimia nervosa. *Behavioural Analysis and Modification* 4: 314-17 (1981).

27. Crisp, A.H.: Anorexia nervosa at normal body weight. The abnormal normal weight control syndrome. *International Journal of Psychiatry in Medicine* 11: 203-33 (1981).

28. Pyle, R.L., Mitchell, J.E. and Eckert, E.: Bulimia: A report of 34 cases. *Journal of Clinical Psychiatry* 42: 60-4 (1981).

29. Katz, J.L. and Sitnick, T.: Anorexia nervosa and bulimia. *Archives of General Psychiatry* 39: 487-9 (1982).

30. Lucas, A.R.: Pigging out. *Journal of the American Medical Association* 247: 82 (1982).

31. Rost, W., Neuhaus, M. and Florin, I.: Bulimia nervosa – sex role attitude, sex role behaviour, and sex role related locus of control in bulimarexic women. *Journal of Psychosomatic Research* 26: 403-8 (1982).

32. Schwartz, D.M., Thompson, M.G. and Johnson, C.L.: Anorexia nervosa and bulimia: The sociocultural context. *International Journal of Eating Disorders* 1: 20-36 (1982).

33. Garner, D.M., Olmstead, M.P. and Garfinkel, P.E.: Does anorexia nervosa occur on a continuum? *International Journal of Eating Disorders* 2: 11-20 (1983).

34. Huon, G.F. and Brown, L.B.: Bulimia: the emergence of a syndrome. *Australian and New Zealand Journal of Psychiatry* 18: 113-26 (1984).

35. Fairburn, C.G. and Cooper, P.J.: Self-induced vomiting and bulimia nervosa: an undetected problem. *British Medical Journal 284: 1153-5 (1982).*

36. Huon, G.F.: An initial validation of a self-help program for Bulimia. *International Journal of Eating Disorders* 1985 (in press).

37. Secord, P.F. and Jourard, S.M.: The appraisal of body-cathexis. Body cathexis and the self. *Journal of Consulting Psychology*17: 343-7 (1953).

38. Abrahams, S.F. and Beumont, P.J.V.: How patients describe bulimia or binge eating. *Psychological Medicine* 12: 625-35 (1982).

39. Johnson, C., Connors, M. and Stuckey, M.: Short term group treatment of bulimia. *International Journal of Eating Disorders* 2: 199-208 (1983).

40. Moss, R.A., Prue, D.M., Lomax, D. and Martin, J.E.: Implications of self-monitoring for smoking treatment: effects on adherence and session attendance. *Addictive Behaviour* 7: 381-5 (1983).

41. Norman, D.K. and Herzog, D.B.: Bulimia, anorexia nervosa, and anorexia nervosa with bulimia – a comparative analysis of MMPI profiles. *International Journal of Eating Disorders* 2: 43-52 (1983).

Chapter VIII

The Treatment of Bulimia

Bulimia has only recently been described as a discrete clinical entity.[1-3]

Not all workers in this area agree on diagnostic criteria for bulimia, [3] but among the most commonly used criteria are those of the American Psychiatric Association, which are:

A. Recurrent episodes of binge eating (rapid consumption of a large amount of food in a discrete period of time, usually less than 2 hours).

B. At least 3 of the following:
  1. consumption of high-caloric, easily ingested food during a binge;
  2. inconspicuous eating during a binge;
  3. termination of such eating episodes by abdominal pain, sleep, social interruption, or self-induced vomiting;
  4. repeated attempts to lose weight by severely restrictive diets, self-induced vomiting, or use of cathartics or diuretics;
  5. frequent weight fluctuations greater than 4.5kg due to alternating binges and fasts.

C. Awareness that the eating pattern is abnormal and fear of not being able to stop eating voluntarily.

D. Depressed mood and self-depreciative thoughts following eating binges.

E. The bulimic episodes are not due to anorexia nervosa or any known physical disorder.

Essentially, the disorder is characterized by episodes of eating large amounts of food for which the patient attempts to compensate by the use of weight-losing behaviour such as starvation, induced vomiting, or purgation. These episodes are perceived by the patient as being beyond her conscious control. The patient is usually preoccupied with body weight and shape, and the control of these.

Bulimia appears to be a common problem amongst young women in Western society.[4-6] It is estimated that perhaps as many as 20% of young women experience episodes of binge-eating which they feel is beyond their conscious control. Since recent publicity in the popular press, many of these women now seek professional help for their eating disorder.

Opinions vary as to the optimal management approach to bulimia, and since the disorder has only recently been described in a systematic fashion, long-term outcome studies are rare. This paper presents the general principles used in our unit to manage these problems; our approach is similar to that of Fairburn.[7]

Assessment

Assessment is the first and perhaps most important step in the management of bulimia. It is necessary to detect and treat any life-threatening complications of the disorder as soon as possible. Assessment also clarifies for the patient, as well as the therapist, the nature of the eating problem, the pattern of the behaviour, and allows both parties to set goals and priorities for management. It is also important to have a clear record of the clinical picture at presentation, not only to be able to provide appropriate treatment but also to be able to assess outcome and progress at follow-up.

Assessment, as well as ongoing management, requires a team approach. The team should include a therapist who deals with the psychological aspects of bulimia and a physician aware of the physical complications of the behaviours used by patients with bulimia for attempted weight control. The team may require access to other health professionals, such as dietitians, social workers, and gynaecologists.

Interview

At first attendance at our unit the therapist who is to be responsible for the ongoing management of the patient's psychological problems conducts an interview to:

1. Obtain a detailed description of the behaviours, psychopathology and events causing the patient distress;[2]
2. Establish the duration of the condition;
3. Obtain a detailed history of the factors which preceded and were associated with the onset of disordered eating;
4. Obtain a detailed history of those factors which may be associated with the continuation of the disordered eating, determine how and to what extent the eating disorder interferes with the patient's life;
5. Assess the risk of suicide.

Medical Consultation

The medical consultation is carried out by a practitioner other than the therapist. This allows direct and often 'invasive' questioning which may otherwise jeopardize the psychotherapeutic relationship. The medical consultation includes:

1. Medical history – including a general history and a history of abnormal eating behaviours, as well as specific questioning on symptoms resulting from these abnormal behaviours. The patient should be asked about the use of diuretics, abuse of purgatives, self-induced vomiting (and means of inducing vomiting), excessive exercise for weight control, starvation and the use of 'social' drugs such as alcohol. Symptoms resulting from pathological disturbances consequent upon these behaviours are also sought specifically. For example, frequent muscle cramps during the waking hours and paraesthesia suggest that the patient may have a metabolic alkalosis secondary to self-induced vomiting.[8]. A gynaecological history should also be taken, including questions about the method of contraception used by the patient. This provides an opportunity for the physician to discuss such issues as fertility, and the need for contraception even if a sexually active patient has amenorrhoea, as menstrual cycles can resume unexpectedly as the patient's treatment progresses.

2. Physical examination to exclude clinically detectable illness; Trousseau's sign is useful if alkalosis is suspected.

3. Laboratory investigations – all patients at our unit have blood taken for estimation of sodium, potassium, chloride, total carbon dioxide, creatinine and urea levels and a full blood count.

Many of the physical complications of binge eating and associated behaviours are serious, and further investigations are ordered as required, e.g. an electrocardiograph may be indicated if a hypochloraemic hypokalaemic alkalosis is detected.[8]

The physician conducting the medical assessment is also able to inform the patient of the possible consequences of their behaviours and is usually able to reassure the patient that she has not as yet caused irreversible damage to her body.

Management

Bulimia requires an eclectic approach from the therapist. It is difficult to give a precise plan of management for a problem that occurs in people of varied backgrounds, ages and social circumstance, and that appears to be so common. Some general principles do emerge, however, and these are discussed below. Bulimia, more than many other disorder, requires a flexible, tolerant therapist, who is prepared to innovate and to 'tailor' a treatment plan to individual patients.

However, we would like to stress that one of the most important factors in the outcome of treatment is the patient's motivation to change.[9] Where the patient is diffident or even hostile at the suggestion that the established habits of behaviour and thinking will have to change, the treatment is unlikely to be successful. At times the therapist may play a supportive role until the patient is 'ready' to 'get better' or has made changes in her lifestyle which allow her to modify her behaviour, such as resolving marital conflicts. Thus, treatment initiated by the patient carries a greater chance of a favourable outcome than treatment initiated by concerned friends and relatives.

Aims

The aims of therapy are for the patient to:[9]
1. acquire new attitudes to food and weight;
2. control weight;
3. avoid inappropriate methods of losing weight;
4. recognize a 'bad mood';
5. recognize what precipitates binge-eating;
6. find ways of coping with problems, other than resorting to binge-eating.

The overall aim is to enable the patient to live a reasonably normal life and cope without professional support. Many will need assistance to develop the skills and confidence necessary to cope with everyday adult life. This maturing process is often a long and uneven one, but some of the intermediate aims can be achieved in a shorter time.

Our approach is similar to the 'cognitive behavioural' approach of Fairburn, where the role of the therapist is to 'provide information, advice and support'.[7]

Management of eating and weight control behaviours is conducted on an outpatient basis. Hospital admission is to be avoided as experience has shown that improvement after inpatient treatment is no better than after outpatient treatment[9] and in our experience, some women with eating disorders take on the role of the psychiatric patient following admission to hospital and then manipulate the psychiatric hospital system, seeking readmission with any new stress. Hospital admission for reasons other than eating and weight control behaviours may be necessary in 3 situations:
1. when the risk of suicide is considered high;
2. when life-threatening medical complications are detected;
3. when the eating behaviour is a symptom of another condition which requires admission for treatment, for example, schizophrenia.

During outpatient treatment it is important that the patient knows there is 24-hour contact with one of the team to provide prompt intervention in the crises to which such patients are prone.

Counselling

The most useful introduction to treatment is providing information to the patient
about her presenting problems. This begins during the initial interview. The therapist should be prepared to provide information about the following:
1. normal eating and weight-losing behaviours, such as, most young women diet,
experience binge-eating and want to weigh less than they do;[4]
2. the risks and complications of bulimia with emphasis on what symptoms need
urgent attention, for example blood in the vomitus; patients should also be aware
that some symptoms may appear transiently when weight controlling behaviours
cease, for example abdominal bloating and constipation may follow ceassation
of laxitive abuse;
3. nutritional aspects including the need to eat something at least 3 times a day
and general discussion on dietary requirements to permit clarification of any
misconceptions about quantity or content of foods;
4. what is a realistic target weight for a given height and age, and what is a
realistic expectation for the patient, including a discussion of the importance of
body fat, and the concept that weight will fluctuate within a couple of kilograms.

Against this educational background the possibility of the patient modifying
her behaviour can be explored and discussed, the aim being to minimize the
preoccupation with weight and eating as soon as possible. All dieting efforts
should cease. Daily weighing, calorie counting, skipping meals, and other techniques often used by young women in their attemps to control weight[4] are discouraged. A sensible dietary pattern which is appropriate to their lifestyle is sub-
stituted for the previous chaos, and it may also be useful to borrow some of the
techniques used in management of obesity (for example, suggesting that all food
be consumed sitting down, at a set table). The advice of a dietitian may be
requested at this point. Patients should be discouraged from taking employment
that involves dealing with food throughout their working day, though this is often
difficult, particularly for patients requiring part-time work.

The fact that alcohol and marijuana may impair impulse control is usually
recognized by the patients. Next, the therapist should explore the patterns of
binge-eating with the patient. Identification of precipitating factors may be difficult at first, but a food and event record is often helpful.[7] The patient and
therapist work together to identify points at which intervention can abort the
impending binge, and develop pleasurable alternatives to substitute at the necessary moment. It is wise to have several alternatives; alternatives that have
some motor activity involved and that occupy the hands or mouth (e.g. knitting,
washing hair, talking to a friend on the telephone) are often more effective. Most
patients are prepared to alter their daily routine to prevent binge-prone circumstances. If, for example, binge-eating is particularly likely on arrival home from
work, stopping off at a gym for an exercise class may provide a distraction.

Some patients will benefit from instruction in relaxation techniques at some time during the course of therapy. With practice a relaxation technique (whichever the patient enjoys) may be used as a substitute for binge-eating. Relaxation, if used regularly, also conveys general benefits, such as the general reduction of anxiety and tension which, in itself, may help prevent binge-eating episodes. Relaxation is often seen by the patient to be more useful later in treatment when the frequency of binge-eating and associated behaviours has been reduced or has ceased. With time, the therapist can provide some insight into the function of the eating disorder for the patient. Discussion of events and moods surrounding the onset of the binge are often a source of understanding for the patient. Taking a broader view, and examining the general events surrounding the exacerbations of the disorder in the past will often reveal how the disorder has been 'used' by the patient to avoid conflict or stress, for example, the use of bulimia to provide a 'moratorium' on sexual activity.[9] Gaining insight into the 'advantages' of the behaviour can be reassuring to the patient who is frustrated by the failure of previous cures. The patient's ideas concerning the importance of appearance, body weight and shape should also be addressed. The patient can be encouraged to find other, more durable, sources of self-worth. It is striking how often bulimic patients display a rather concrete, 'all or nothing' style of thinking,[7] and they seem to continue the 'magical' thinking of childhood. This is perhaps best displayed in their selection of dieting methods – instant cures and overnight success are especially attractive.[4] These issues will need to be addressed at some time during therapy and an attempt made to help the patient develop a more mature style of problem-solving.

During the course of therapy, as the eating problem resolves, other problems, often age-related, will emerge.[9] These may be conflicts between the patient and her parents over issues of independence, marital problems, or problems with employment or study. The therapist needs to provide support through these periods, and reassure the patient that any relapse is understandable under the circumstances. It will sometimes be necessary to involve other professionals at this point, for example, a marriage counsellor. It is these problems which usually play the biggest part in therapy.

It is important that the therapist can provide reassurance and at all times assist in improving the patient's self-esteem. Thought-blocking techniques may be useful. Many patients' expectations of themselves are impractical in the time span they set. Recognition of small day-to-day achievements and the development of self-worth are essential in treatment.

Medication

Many bulimic patients use or abuse substances at some time during their lives. They are also known to be at high risk of suicide.[1] For this reason we recommend that any medication be prescribed for these patients with great caution. It should also be remembered that some of the preparations used by bulimic patients in their attempts to control weight are available 'over the counter' (though this does not mean they are harmless),[10] and the patient may be using such drugs without confiding in her therapist, so drug interaction may be a problem.

The following specific medications have been considered for use in the management of bulimia.

There is no evidence that appetite suppressants are of any value in the management of bulimia, many patients having taken these before presenting for treatment. Rather, there are theoretical reasons for avoiding them, since one of the aims of therapy is to give the patient confidence in her own control of eating, and in the long term allow her to rediscover the feelings of hunger and satiation.

Psychotropic medication may be considered for use as an adjunct to therapy, where the individual patient's psychopathology requires it. Caution should be exercised as patients may consume large amounts of a drug with sedating effects in order to prevent themselves bingeing. Tricyclic antidepressants are potentially lethal in large doses, and even in prescribed doses may exert a cardiac irritant effect.[11] Toxicity is increased in the presence of hypokalaemia and alkalosis, producing potentially fatal cardiac arrhythmias. Nevertheless, there are some theoretical grounds for advocating the use of antidepressants in bulimia,[12] and some encouraging results have been reported from some centres in selected patients.[12] We reserve these drugs for a sub-group of patients whose clinical picture includes strong elements of depression, and who are quite reliable.

Monoamine-oxidase inhibitors are contra-indicated, as bulimic patients are unlikely to be able to comply with the dietary restrictions necessary.

Lithium poses problems because the levels in circulating blood can vary markedly with renal function and sodium level (which may be altered by diuretic abuse). Renal function may deteriorate rapidly in bulimia.[11]

Benzodiazepines, while relatively safe, may be taken in excess for their sedative effect. Beta-blockers, also used to reduce anxiety symptoms, may increase the risk of cardiac arrhythmia if alkalosis is present, by increasing heart block via its action on the rate of conduction at the A-V node.[13]

Dietary supplements may be deemed necessary to correct a deficiency state, for example, iron supplements in those with demonstrated iron deficiency.

Finally, bulimia sufferers may require medication for intercurrent illnesses during the treatment of their bulimia. It is sometimes possible for these agents to increase pathology due to bulimia. For example, mefenamic acid, taken to relieve menstrual cramps, may increase gastric blood loss by exacerbating vomiting-related gastritis.

Over the last 2 decades an increasing amount of attention has been directed towards the eating disorders. Although bulimia is only recently described as a clinical entity, it has attracted a great deal of attention both in the lay press and within the academic literature. Treatment approaches are being adapted for use in these patients, and self-help groups have emerged in major cities. Elsewhere in this book Huon reports on her development of an innovative mail-order treatment programme for bulimia sufferers.

In 1983 Lacey reported on the use of a combination of individual psychotherapy and group psychotherapy, over a 10-week course.[14] At follow-up, 2 years later, 20 out of 30 patients reported 'no bulimic or vomiting episodes'. In a study of outcome conducted at our unit in 1982 we reviewed 43 patients 1 to 5 years after treatment.[15] At interview assessment 40% were judged to be 'cured' (ie. bodyweight stable within 3 kilograms, binge-eating episodes less than once a month, no self-induced vomiting, no laxative use, no dieting). A further 31% had modified their behaviour sufficiently to be considered 'improved' (ie, binge-eating, self-induced vomiting and laxative use all occurred less than once per week, weight was stable and any dieting conducted used 'sensible' methods).

There is a need for the development of acceptable and objective measures of outcome. Currently there is little agreement between the different methods used; for example, self-report, interview and questionnaire.[16] Two measures which appear to offer promise are EVA (described elsewhere in this book) and the EDI.[16]

The current outcome results are certainly encouraging for both patient and therapist. As the condition is better understood, and the diagnostic criteria are refined, assessment of outcome will also change, hopefully for the better.

References

1. Russell, G.: Bulimia nervosa: an ominous variant of anorexia nervosa, *Psychological Medicine* 9: 429-38 (1979).
2. Abraham, S.F. and Beumont, P.J.V.: How patients describe bulimia or binge eating. *Psychological Medicine* 12: 625-35 (1982).
3. American Psychiatric Association: *Diagnostic and Statistical Manual of Mental Disorders,* 3rd ed. (APA, Washington DC 1980).
4. Abraham, S.F., Mira, M., Beumont, P.J.V., Sowerbutts, T.D. and Llewellyn-Jones, D.: Eating behaviours among young women. *Medical Journal of Australia* 2: 225-8 (1983).
5. Halmi, K.A., Falk, J.R. and Schwartz, E.: Binge-eating and vomiting: a survey of college population. *Psychological Medicine* 11: 697-706 (1981).
6. Cooper, P.J. and Fairburn, C.G.: Binge-eating and self-induced vomiting in the community: a preliminary study. *British Journal Psychiatry* 142: 139-44 (1983).
7. Fairburn, C.G.: Bulimia: its epidemiology and management; in: Stunkard and Steller (Eds) *Eating and Its Disorders* (Raven Press, New York 1984).
8. Mira, M., Stewart, P. and Abraham, S.F.: Hypokalaemia and renal impairment in patients with eating disorders. *Medical Journal of Australia* 140: 290-2 (1984).
9. Abraham, S.F. and Llewellyn-Jones, D.: *Eating Disorders: the Facts.* (Oxford University Press, Oxford 1984).
10. Dobb, G.J. and Edis, R.H.: Coma and neuropathy after ingestion of herbal laxative containing podophyllum. *Medical Journal of Australia* 140: 495-6 (1984).

11. Badessarine, R.J.: Drugs in the treatment of psychiatric disorders; in Goodman, Goodman and Gilman (Eds) *The Pharmacological Basis of Therapeutics*. 6th ed (MacMillian Co. New York 1980).

12. Hudson, J.I., Pope, H.G. and Jonas, J.M.: Treatment of Bulimia with antidepressants: theoretical considerations and clinical findings; in Stunkard and Stellar (Eds) *Eating and Its Disorders* (Raven Press, New York 1984).

13. Bigger, J.J. and Haffman, B.F.: Antiarrhythmic drugs; in Goodman, Goodman and Gilman (Eds) *The Pharmacological Basis of Therapeutics*. 6th ed (MacMillian Co. New York 1980).

14. Lacey, J.H.: Bulimia nervosa, binge-eating and psychogenic vomiting: a controlled treatment study and long-term outcome. *British Medical Journal* 286: 1609-13 (1983).

15. Abraham, S.F., Mira, M. and Llewellyn-Jones, D.: Bulimia A Study of Outcome. *International Journal of Eating Disorders* 2 (4): 175-80 (1983).

16. Garner, D.M., Olmstead, M.P. and Polivy, J.: Development and Validation of a Multidimensional Eating Disorder Inventory for Anorexia Nervosa and Bulimia. *International Journal of Eating Disorders* 2 (2): 15-34 (1983).

Chapter IX

Epidemiology of Obesity

There is no meaning in statements of the type 'x% of people in Australia are obese'. The figure and its interpretation depend on:
1. the type of people;
2. the time in history when the sample was examined;
3. the place in which the sample is collected;
4. the method used to measure obesity;
5. the definition and standards chosen for obesity and overweight;
6. the degree of obesity or overweight.

Since there have been very few national samples examined for obesity in different countries, it is likewise usually impossible to substantiate impressions like 'there are more fat people in Eastern Europe than India' or 'people are fatter nowadays than they used to be'.

Age

Infants who are not breast-fed are susceptible to overweight because they need to drink but have no control over the calorie density of the drinks they are given. Figures for the prevalence of obesity in infants depend on the proportion predominantly breast-fed; older figures on infantile obesity are no longer applicable since breast-feeding is more widespread. Obesity is uncommon once toddlers start running around.

School children who are unable to exercise for some medical reason can become overweight. Nowadays 3 factors may be reducing the exercise that children get and thus tending to produce a more overweight generation: the danger of cycling to school; urban overcrowding and discontinuation of compulsory games at school; and the number of hours children spend watching television (hours when they might otherwise be more active). In South Australia daily exercise periods have been introduced (? reintroduced) to many primary schools. In preliminary studies the school exercise programme led to less overweight children and improved academic performance.

Activity and food intake among adolescents varies greatly. Some exercise hard each day, training for or playing in competitive sport and then dance all night. Other adolescents become entirely sedentary and are able to use a parental car instead of their legs to visit friends.

Some figures of Court's from Victoria give a general idea of numbers. At least 3% of young children in Australia are obese[1] and among secondary school students (aged 11 to 18 years) 8% of girls weigh more than 20% above expected weight for height and from 3.5% to 6% of boys, increasing with age.[2]

In adults the prevalence of obesity is relatively low in the 20 to 25 year age group and then in industrial societies it rises fast into middle age. Giving up participant sport in men and accumulation of fat with each pregnancy in women are important contributors to the middle-age spread. Note that this occurs at a younger age than many people think of as middle aged (Table 1). In old people there is less obesity and mean weights (for height) decline. Lean body mass shrinks slowly from middle age [3] and there is selective loss of obese people who have higher-than-expected mortalities from several diseases. The middle-age spread is not seen universally, for example, not in hunter-gatherers.[4]

Sex

Usually there is more obesity in females, especially in adolescence and in middle age. Even at similar weights for height women have a higher proportion of adipose tissue in their bodies – about 26% compared with 12% in men.[5] Oestrogens favour fat deposition and androgens favour muscle.

In parts of Africa plump women are desired by men and admired by their sisters and, provided food is available, there are nearly as many fat women in their late 20s as in middle age. [6] Deliberate fattening of women for marriage still persists in places.[7]

On the other hand, in sophisticated Western cities, the fashionable shape for women, as can be seen on the covers of fashion magazines,[8] has been slender for most of this century, especially in the 1920s and 1960s and the generalization that women are more likely to be obese than men no longer applies [3] (Table 1).

Epidemiology of obesity

Table 1. Australian National Heart Foundation: Risk Factor·Prevalence Study 1980 Quetelet body mass index – W/H² in kg/m².* The W/H² cut-offs used were: men – underweight < 19, overweight 26 to 30, obese > 30; women – underweight < 18, overweight 25 to 30, obese > 30.

All cities	25-29 years	30-34 years	35-39 years	40-44 years	45-49 years	50-54 years	55-59 years	60-64 years	All ages
Male†									
Column percentages	100.0	100.0	100.0	100.0	100.0	100.0	100.0	100.0	100.0
Underweight	4.5	3.5	3.0	3.4	2.9	1.4	1.0	1.9	2.9
Acceptable weight	65.8	68.6	51.1	49.7	45.1	54.5	47.9	51.3	55.7
Overweight	26.7	22.9	40.6	36.9	42.9	34.3	40.3	37.4	34.1
Obese	3.1	4.9	5.4	10.0	9.1	9.7	10.8	9.4	7.2
Weighted mean	24	25	26	26	26	26	26	26	26
5th centile	20	20	20	21	20	21	21	20	20
Median	23	24	25	25	26	25	26	25	25
95th centile	30	30	31	32	32	32	32	32	31
Female ‡ §									
Column percentages	100.0	100.0	100.0	100.0	100.0	100.0	100.0	100.0	100.0
Underweight	11.2	7.3	5.9	5.5	4.5	3.6	2.6	2.7	5.9
Acceptable weight	74.5	71.5	71.3	57.2	58.8	53.1	53.3	46.8	62.6
Overweight	13.0	17.4	13.5	30.9	28.5	32.1	34.7	39.1	24.5
Obese	1.3	3.8	9.3	6.3	8.1	11.2	9.5	11.3	7.0
Weighted mean	22	23	24	24	25	25	25	25	24
5th centile	18	18	18	18	19	19	19	19	18
Median	21	22	22	23	23	24	24	25	23
95th centile	28	29	33	31	33	35	32	33	32

* One kilogram was deducted from the measured weight, as a correction for the weight of clothing, in computation of the body mass index.
† Total n=2765.
‡ Excludes pregnant women. § n=2785.

Occupation

In some jobs obesity is traditionally thought to be an occupational hazard – cooks and barmen, for example. But most master chefs that I have seen in photographs or on TV have not been fat. Perhaps there is a social class effect (see below) operating here as well. Sumo wrestlers are perhaps the archetype of occupational obesity. In other occupations obesity is unacceptable and not seen – fashion models, ballet dancers, jockeys and aircrew. This phenomenon is probably also becoming widespread among dietitians.

Table 2. Prevalence of obesity in ethnic groups.

Ethnic Group	Per cent obese by socio-economic status		
	Low	Medium	High
American (4th generation)	13	4	4
Russian, Polish, Lithuanian	18	12	10
British	23	0	10
Irish	25	16	3
Italian	32	23	-*
German, Austrian	35	16	4
Czechoslovakian	41	92	-*
Hungarian	44	24	-*

* Numbers per cell insufficient.

Social Class

In the least-developed Third World countries fat and even sleek people can only be found in the ruling and merchant minorities of the population. But in affluent countries the social class gradient is reversed. There is more obesity in the poor, [9,10] in children as well as adults. [11]

Ethnic Group

In New Zealand the Maoris show more obesity than the whites. [12] In countries like the USA and Australia where there are many immigrants from different parts of the world, there are obvious differences in the prevalence of obesity. It is necessary to correct for socio-economic status. Table 2 shows an example from the USA.[13]

In Australia, Rutishauser and Hunter reported an excess of obese children of Italian origin among 6-year olds in Geelong.[14]

Smoking

If people give up smoking they commonly put on some weight. [15] Smoking tends to suppress appetite and may increase resting metabolic rate. [16] Smokers on the average weigh less than non-smokers. [17,18] This affects mortality at weights for height below the acceptable (or desirable) range. If smokers are removed, the excess mortality which is recorded at this zone of the scale is reduced. [19]

Era

It is often loosely said in the media that the prevalence of obesity is increasing. There are seldom enough figures, using the same methods and criteria, for comparisons of generations to be made. Young women today in Western cities are probably thinner than their mothers and grandmothers were at the same age. In Framingham 5-year cohorts of women born in the first 20 years of this century have become progressively lighter in middle age [3] but in the same period the men have become heavier. In Britain, too, men entering the Army became heavier from 1952 to 1972.[20]

In the only Australian publication on this that I have seen, Dugdale *et al.* compared heights and weights of schoolchildren in Queensland from 1911 with measurements in 1950 and 1976. [21] Weights for age increased. In boys this was proportional to increased stature but in girls there appears to have been an increase in weight for height.

Place Where Sample Is Collected

People can be collected for examination in 3 broad ways.
1. At the workplace, e.g., a large firm, factory or office block and from routine examinations in the armed forces or at school. This is a convenient way of collecting a sample and the best way of studying children of school-going age. But for adults the sample leaves out other members of the family and people in other occupations.
2. By self-referral, e.g., those taking out life insurance or those concerned about their health who go to a clinic for health examination. The data in Table 3 come from a coronary risk factor screening programme which was set up in a large department store and offered a limited free examination for interested people. It presumably contains a concentration of people worried about or interested in their health. Table 4 comes from a fee-paying health examination centre which provides a comprehensive series of tests and is likely to contain an over-representation of the more affluent adults in Sydney.
3. Some sort of community sample is the ideal method but it is more expensive and time-consuming. The data in Table 1 were obtained in this way from random sampling of the electoral roll in Sydney north, Sydney south, Melbourne, Brisbane, Adelaide, Perth and Hobart. It is very near to a national sample except

that it omits rural residents and people without fixed addresses. The overall response rate was 76%.

Table 3. Weight classification of 10 000 self-referred people Sydney 1976-77.[34]

Relative body weight*	Age (years)					
	21 to 39		40 to 59		60 +	
	men	women	men	women	men	women
> 110%	33%	19.5%	44%	36%	37%	41%
> 120%	12%	9.5%	17%	16%	13%	20%
> 130%	4%	4%	6%	8%	5%	8%

* Based on medium frame.

Table 4. Weights of female and male subjects in relation to their 'desirable' weight for height.[35]

Age group (years)	Percentage of subjects whose weight is:							
	More than 10% below 'desirable' weight		Within ± 10% of 'desirable' weight		More than 10% above 'desirable' weight		Number of subjects	
	Females	Males	Females	Males	Females	Males	Females	Males
20-24	24	12	63	64	13	24	1745	1493
25-29	21	7	64	57	15	36	2765	3935
30-34	15	4	65	52	20	44	3298	5696
35-39	12	3	64	46	24	51	3459	5598
40-49	7	3	59	42	34	55	7856	11553
50-59	6	3	53	39	41	58	7609	9076
60-69	7	4	49	40	44	56	3234	3589
Over 70	9	6	48	47	43	47	543	567
							30509	41507

Source : Medicheck Referral Centre (February 1973 to December 1978).

Method Used to Measure Obesity

Obesity is an excess of body fat [3] or adipose tissue. The commonest method for measuring it, by *weighing people,* is indirect. Body weight can be increased by oedema, increased muscular development, and large bones as well as heavy clothes. The weight has to be read against height, which is not an easy measurement to take exactly [22] and almost impossible if the subject has a deformity like kyphoscoliosis or arthritis of both knees.

Of the other methods, skinfold thickness – 1 or the sum of 2 or 4 – is the only other technique simple enough for use with large numbers of people. Disadvantages of skinfolds include inter-observer error, ethnic differences in the distribution of subcutaneous fat and the impossibility of obtaining measurements on very obese people. [23]

Underwater weighing; counting ^{40}K; uptake of a fat-soluble gas like xenon, etc., are expensive research techniques. Their only use is for validation of the quicker techniques.

Definition and Standards

Adults

There are 2 criteria for deciding whether someone is too fat. One is social or fashion, 'I'm too fat to fit this season's dresses', and there are plenty of women in affluent communities who are dieting but not overweight in medical terms. Their criterion for obesity is aesthetic and subjective.

The other criterion is actuarial and objective: at what weight for height is the (age standardized) risk of dying at its lowest? How should life insurance premiums be loaded for people above (or below) the acceptable range of weight for height? This, of course, is the scientific, medical and epidemiological way of defining obesity. On a plot of mortality against weight for height, obesity starts when the mortality curve turns clearly upwards from the trough of lowest mortality at 'acceptable' or 'desirable' weight.

The accepted way of expressing weight for height when working with group data is

$$\frac{\text{weight (kg)}}{\text{height (m)}^2}$$

the body-mass index or Quetelet's index [24] because it is largely independent of height. For individual patients tables of weight for height are more convenient.

Table 5. 'Normal' weight standards for adults.

	For persons 168cm tall without shoes		
	kg Men	kg Women	Notes
Metropolitan Life Insurance Co. New York 1959 'desirable' [25] weights	55 to 70	53 to 68	Bottom of small frame to top of large frame, original .converted to metric; 2.5 and 5cm taken off for shoes and 3 and 2kg for clothes from men and women.
Fogarty Conference 1975 [26]	56 to 71	52 to 66	Ranges of recommended weights converted to metric (no shoes or clothes).
W/H^2 (kg/m^2) 20 to 25	56 to 71	56 to 71	Adopted by Garrow [28]
Metropolitan Life Insurance Co. New York 1983 [29]	60 to 74	54 to 73	Bottom of small frame to top of large frame. Weights with lowest mortality. One inch from heights of men and women, 5lbs for clothes from men, 3lbs from women, then converted to kg.

For adults 4 different *standards* in use or proposed at present are compared in Table 5 for a height of 168cm.

1. The 'desirable' weights of the Metropolitan Life Insurance Co. of New York (1959) [25] are still the principal standard in use. They are based on actuarial experience of persons examined for life insurance in the USA between 1935 and 1953. They are usually presented as 3 ranges for arbitrary small, medium and large frame sizes. At 168cm height (without shoes) these are: small frame 55 to 59kg; medium frame 58 to 64kg and large frame 61 to 70kg (for men) unclothed.

They were originally published with heights in feet and inches but wearing shoes, weight in pounds and wearing indoor clothing (including shoes). Some subsequent versions have converted them to metric units and/or taken off 2.5cm for men's shoes and 5cm for women's and/or have taken off 3kg for men's clothes and 2kg for the weight of women's clothes. As a result tables printed in books vary.

2. The Fogarty Conference [26] was an international meeting held at the National Institutes of Health, Bethesda, Maryland, USA, in 1973. It adopted a simplified version of the Metropolitan Life Insurance Co.'s desirable weights but without shoes or clothes. This standard has been used in the USA and in the 1983 Royal College of Physicians' Obesity Report. [19]

3. In effect, the acceptable range of weights in the Fogarty standard corresponds to W/H^2 of 20 to 25 in men and 18.7 to 23.8 in women. Use of W/H^2 enables the disease experience for all heights to be plotted together against bodyweight. Recent data, however, from large prospective studies [27] not confined to persons taking life insurance do not show mortality increasing at lower W/H^2 in women than in men. Indeed, there is some evidence that lower segment, gynoid type of obesity has a lower risk for hypertension and diabetes. [28] Garrow has adopted a unisex W/H^2 ratio for grading obesity in his book.[29] It has the merit of simplicity.*

4. The 1983 weights with lowest mortality from the Metropolitan Life Insurance Co. [30] are higher than their earlier desirable weights. They are based on the 1979 Build and Blood Pressure Study of the Society of Actuaries. They have not yet been accepted by health authorities.

Obesity is usually taken as starting in adults 20% above the desirable or acceptable weight. The big question has been which normal weight? Some workers have used the mid-weight of the medium frame desirable weights and then added 20% but it is recommended both by the Fogarty Conference [26] and in the British DHSS/MRC report [20] that for public health work the 20% should be added on to the top end of large frame desirable weights – in other words the upper end of the range of acceptable weights for each particular height. This is at a W/H^2 of approximately 25, so that obesity starts at a W/H^2 of 30. And follow-up studies show increases in mortality and morbidity above W/H^2 of 30.

Figures of the prevalence of obesity are confusing because they have used different standards. In Table 3 the normal was taken as the desirable weight for medium frame. This means that 120% relative bodyweight is less than if the upper end of desirable weights for large frame had been used. Likewise the normal for Table 4 appears to have been somewhere in the middle of the range of desirable weights. Ten per cent added to this represents only mild overweight, not obesity. In Table 1 obesity starts at a W/H^2 of 30. This is now generally thought to be the standard cut-off for obesity (it is a higher weight than 120% in Table 3). Table 1, therefore, not only comes from multiple Australian cities, with random sampling of all settled adult electors, but also has a cut-off for obesity that is biologically meaningful. It can be seen that there is more obesity in men than in women up to the age of 25 years. By 40 to 44 years 10% of men are obese and its prevalance stays about this level until 64 years. In women the top prevalence of obesity is reached 10 years later. The earlier peak of obesity in men has been noted elsewhere. [20] Unfortunately, this survey did not look at people above 65 years of age.

---

* At its October 1984 meeting the National Health and Medical Research Council resolved to adopt W/H^2 of 20 to 25 as the reference standard or acceptable bodyweight for Australian adults. There is at present no recommended single reference level for children in Australia.

Children

Although sampling adults is difficult and results are confusingly reported against different standards, with care they can be meaningful and comparable. In children the diagnosis of obesity is more uncertain. At its worst an investigator uses the percentile standards of weight for age (or weight for height) and may take obesity as starting at the 90th or 95th percentile. He then reports that about 10% or 5% of children (respectively) were found to be obese! No biological risk has been associated with any of the percentiles of the weight standards for children. Dugdale [31] has discussed the alternative method of classifying children >20% above the 50th percentile as obese, just as children weighing <80% of the 50th percentile are usually classified as having mild protein-energy malnutrition. [32] This 20% above median was the criterion used by Court [2] and by Rutishauser, [14] both discussed above. It follows a similar principle to the cut-offs for adult obesity. Nevertheless, it may be more correct to describe a child 20% above median normal weight as 'overweight' rather than 'obese'. [19] The anthropometric reference weights for children now favoured by WHO are the NCHS figures [33] which are based on larger, more modern samples than the Boston (Harvard) or Tanner or NSW (NHMRC) surveys. [22]

Quantitation of obesity in adolescents is even more difficult because of the range of ages at which the adolescent growth spurt starts. There is no accepted international reference table. The Royal College of Physicians' Obesity Report [19] gives a 4-page table of average weights at different heights at different ages in adolescence which could be used and then 20% above this considered overweight.

Degree of Obesity

Mortality and morbidity go up progressively from mild through moderate to gross obesity. A description that a particular age, sex, etc., group shows x% obesity is incomplete. Ideally, one would like to see a frequency distribution curve or histogram which plots the frequency of the different steps of W/H^2. Garrow shows 4 such curves together in his book. [28] Samples of employed men and women have small 'tails' below W/H^2 of 20 and above W/H^2 of 30. Members of a slimming club show no one underweight and about half over W/H^2 of 30. At his hospital obesity clinic hardly anyone is below W/H^2 30 and the group ranges up to W/H^2 57. It follows that treatment of obesity is more difficult in a hospital specialist obesity clinic than in a slimming club. Suppose each reports a 35% success rate, the hospital has done a bigger job.

Lastly, one must always keep in mind the other end of the weight-for-height distribution. In children round the world, undernutrition is much more abundant than obesity. In affluent countries anorexia nervosa may be partly a side effect of our social obsession with avoiding obesity in adolescent and young women. Table 4 shows more young women 10% below desirable weight in Sydney than young men and Table 1 similarly shows more than twice as many women as men had a more serious degree of underweight, below W/H^2 of 18. It could be argued that in young women in their 20s in Australian cities underweight is a larger nutritional problem today than obesity.

References

1. Court, J.M.: Obesity in childhood. *Medical Journal of Australia* 1: 888 (1977).
2. Court, J.M., Dunlop, M., Reynolds, M., Russell, J. and Griffiths, L.: Growth and development of fat in adolescent school children in Victoria. Part I. Normal growth values and prevalence of obesity. *Australian Paediatric Journal* 12: 296-303 (1976).
3. Bray, G.A.: *The Obese Patient*. (W.B. Saunders, Philadelphia & London 1976).
4. Truswell, A.S. and Hansen, J.D.L.: Medical research among the !Kung, in Lee and De Vore (Eds) *Kalahari Hunter Gatherers*, p.167 (Harvard University Press, Cambridge 1976).
5. Davidson, S., Passmore, R., Brock, J.F. and Truswell, A.S.: *Human Nutrition and Dietetics*, 7th ed. (Churchill Livingstone, Edinburgh & London 1979).
6. Johnson, T.O.: Prevalence of overweight and obesity among adult subjects of an urban African population sample. *British Journal of Preventive Social Medicine* 24: 105-9 (1970).
7. Fantino, M., Baigts, F., Cabanac, M. and Apfelbaum, M.: Effects of an overfeeding regimen – the affective component of the sweet sensation. *Appetite*, 4: 155-64 (1983).
8. Packer, W.: *The Art of Vogue Covers*. (Octopus Books, London 1980).
9. Garn, S.M., Bailey, S.M., Cole, P.E. and Higgins, I.T.T.: Level of education, level of income and level of fatness in adults. *American Journal of Clinical Nutrition* 30: 721-5 (1977).
10. Silverstone, T.J., Gordon, R.P. and Stunkard, A.J.: Social factors in obesity in London. *The Practitioner* 202: 682-8 (1969).
11. Stunkard, A.J., d'Aquili, E., Fox, S. and Filion, R.D.L.: Influence of social class on obesity and thinness in children. *Journal of the American Medical Association* 221: 579-84 (1972).
12. Prior, I.A.M.: The price of civilization. *Nutrition Today* 6: 2 (1971).
13. Stunkard, A.J.: Environment and obesity: recent advances in our understanding of regulation of food intake in man. *Federation Proceedings* 27: 1369 (1968).
14. Rutishauser, I.H.E. and Hunter, S.: The Geelong Study. *Proceedings of the Nutrition Society of Australia* 5: 79-87 (1980).
15. Comstock, G.W. and Stone, R.S.: Changes in body weight and subcutaneous fatness related to smoking habits. *Archives of Environmental Health* 24: 271 (1972).
16. Dallosso, H. and James, W.P.T.: Smoking, food intake and thermogenesis. *XII International Congress of Nutrition, San Diego. Abstracts of papers*, No. 324 (1981).
17. Khosla, T. and Lowe, C.R.: Obesity and smoking habits. *British Medical Journal* 4: 10 (1971).
18. Hawthorne, V.M., Murdock, R.M. and Womersley, J.: Body weight of men and women aged 40-64 years from an urban area in the West of Scotland. *Community Medicine* 1: 229 (1979).
19. Obesity. A report of the Royal College of Physicians (Chairman, Sir Douglas Black). *Journal of the Royal College of Physicians of London* 17: 1-58 (1983).
20. Department of Health and Social Security/Medical Research Council: *Research on Obesity. A Report of the DHSS/MRC Group* (compiled by W.P.T. James). (H.M.Stationery Office, London 1976).
21. Dugdale, A.E., O'Hara, V. and May, G.: Changes in body size and fatness of Australian school-children 1911-1976. *Australian Paediatric Journal* 19: 14-17 (1983).

22. Truswell, A.S.: Anthropometric assessment with heights and weights; in Symposium 'The Assessment of Nutritional Status of the Individual and the Community'. *Transactions of the Menzies Foundation* 3: 56-69 (1981).

23. Garrow, J.S.: Indices of adiposity. *Nutrition Abstracts and Reviews* 53: 697-708 (1983).

24. Quetelet, L.A.J.: *Physique Sociale,* Vol. 2, p.92 (C. Marquardt, Brussels 1869).

25. Metropolitan Life Insurance Company: New weight standards for men and women. *Statistical Bulletin of the Metropolitan Life Insurance Company* 40: 1-4 (1959).

26. Bray, G.A. (Ed.): Obesity in Perspective. A conference sponsored by the John E. Fogarty International Center for Advanced Study in the Health Sciences. National Institutes of Health, Bethesda, Maryland, October 1-3, 1973. *DHEW publication No. NIH 75-708.* (Superintendent of Documents, U.S. Government Printing Office, Washington, D.C. 1975).

27. Lew, E.A. and Garfinkel, L.: Variations in mortality by weight among 750,000 men and women. *Journal of Chronic Diseases,* 32: 563 (1979).

28. Garrow, J.S.: *Treat Obesity Seriously.* (Churchill Livingstone, Edinburgh & London 1981).

29. Kissebah, A.H. *et al.*: Relation of body fat distribution to metabolic complications of obesity. *Journal of Clinical Endocrinology and Metabolism,* 54: 254-60 (1982).

30. News from Metropolitan Life Insurance Co.: *1983 Height and Weight Tables announced.* (Metropolitan Life Insurance Co., New York 1983).

31. Dugdale, A.E.: How obese are Australian children? *Journal of Food and Nutrition* (Australian Commonwealth Department of Health) 39: 132-3 (1982).

32. Food and Agriculture Organization (World Health Organization): Joint Expert Committee on Nutrition, 8th report. *Technical Report Series of the World Health Organization No. 477.* (WHO, Geneva 1971).

33. World Health Organization: A Growth Chart for International Use in Maternal and Child Health Care. *Guidelines for Primary Health Care Personnel* (WHO, Geneva 1978).

34. Simons, L.A. and Jones, A.S.: Coronary risk factor screening programme (Myers Stores). *Medical Journal of Australia* 2: 455 (1978).

35. Grosslight, G.M. and Adena, M.A.: Medicheck man versus Metropolitan man — who carries more weight? *Food and Nutrition Notes and Reviews* 37: 48 (1980).

Chapter X

Obesity – The Metabolic Basis

Obesity is common in our affluent society. It is usually considered to be present when weight is 120% or more of the 'acceptable weight' for an individual's height.[1] Over the last few years considerable interest has been shown in this problem, partly because of changes in the community's 'ideal body image' and its new-found concern with health and fitness, and partly because of the cost and medical consequences of overweight and obesity. The treatment of obesity has become big business and community concern has placed additional stress on those who are obese.

Despite this interest, many aspects of the problem are still unclear. The definition and measurement of obesity are still controversial, being based on data collected from insured persons in the USA between 1935 and 1953, weight being adjusted arbitrarily for clothing and shoes, and where necessary 'estimated' weight was taken. The best tables are probably those from the Society of Actuaries Build Study.[2] These tables take no account of increasing weight with age. This change, and an increasing proportion of the body which is adipose tissue with age, should probably be considered normal. Obesity in children requires though there is considerable evidence that overweight in the young is particularly deleterious to health. However, it should be stated that an obese child is not necessarily an obese adult, though there is an increased risk of permanent obesity occurring.[1]

The exact consequences of obesity are still being debated and researched, and of course the causes of obesity are still unknown. Certain facile statements about 'overeating' are usually made, but it is becoming obvious that obesity is a clinical sign of a heterologous group of causes and stresses, any number of which may combine to produce the final body weight. A simplified list of causes is given in Table 1.

This review will emphasize the endocrine and metabolic basis of obesity to provide a cellular foundation upon which the nutritional and psychological factors which are also important in aetiology can be discussed. We shall not be concerned with 'increased energy ingestion'. Treatment regimes for obesity should be based on consideration of all aetiological factors. Individual differences in metabolism (either primary or secondary) may be important for the development and perpetuation of obesity.

Decreased Energy Expenditure

It is obvious that for any given energy intake (or diet), any decrease in physical activity will result in a gradual weight gain. Changes in activity may be quite

Table 1. Causes of Obesity.

1. *Increased Energy Ingestion*
    a) true hyperphagia – hypothalamic damage
        – altered feedback of metabolic fuels on feeding centre
        – acquired
        – inherited
        – congenital   } e.g. Prader-Willi syndrome
    b) 'relative' hyperphagia – social
        – behavioural
        – psychological

2. *Decreased Energy Expenditure*
    a) altered mobility (decreased activity) – immobilization
        – altered pattern of activity
    b) metabolic changes – diet-induced thermogenesis
        – 'futile cycles'
        – decreased basal metabolic rate
        (e.g. low activity of Na/K ATP'ase)

3. *Endocrine Causes*
    a) Diabetes Mellitus (Type II)
    b) Cushing's Disease – glucocorticoids
    c) Acromegaly
    d) Hypothyroidism
    e) Hypogonadism
    f) Hyperprolactinaemia

subtle, such as changing jobs, a new house, different numbers of people and children in the home, as well as the more obvious ones of giving up regular sport and settling back to enjoy life in front of the television. However, it has been known for years that there are surprising differences in the resting metabolic rate even in individuals of the same surface area, age and sex with similar physical activity.[3] Individuals who can 'eat what they like and not gain weight' are known and widely quoted by obese patients. Also, the body's basal metabolic rate (BMR) alters with changes in energy intake,[4] and this is true of both obese and normal-weight individuals. This decrease in energy expenditure which occurs with strict dieting has led to the concept of 'maximum calorie (subthreshold) diets'[5] in which energy intake is only slightly restricted, aiming to prevent this metabolic adaptation which is detrimental to weight loss.

Studies on obese patients have shown widely varying results, some having low metabolic rates[6] and some surprisingly high rates which indicate that there must be a defect in food intake in these patients.[7] The actual value of the BMR in obese individuals is therefore uncertain and in any case it is difficult to measure, particularly as the 'normal' metabolic rate is always expressed in terms of surface area. It is interesting to note that 2 studies have suggested that formerly obese patients have low BMRs[8] and that children from obese families (considered therefore pre-obese) also have low BMRs.[9]

It must be stated that the value of the BMR in any one obese individual cannot be presumed to be low. However, other possible mechanisms may account for a decreased energy expenditure – 3 of these will be considered.

Diet-induced Thermogenesis

There has been a recent increase in interest in the process whereby individuals are able to maintain their weight despite variable energy ingestion by altering their ability to produce heat. The cellular mechanism of variable heat production is now understood, at least in animals. Rothwell and Stock fed rats on 4 foods each day in addition to their usual rat chow. These extra foods consisted of chocolate chip cookies, sandwiches, potato crisps, cake, Mars bars, etc., and the diet was called 'cafeteria-feeding'. Rats ate the extra foods and continued to eat their usual chow. Each morning uneaten food was removed and the remaining rat chow weighed so that the energy content of the diet eaten could be calculated. Though the 'cafeteria-fed' rats were heavier than age-matched control animals, the weight gain was less than expected considering the increased energy intake. After consuming 80% more energy, weight gain was only 27% greater than that of controls. A source of energy loss was sought in the obese animals. Resting oxygen consumption, a measure of thermogenesis, was increased in the obese animals, as was the amount of brown adipose tissue. It was proposed that this tissue was the source of extra heat production and energy loss.

Brown adipose tissue (BAT) is a highly specialized tissue and is responsible for cold-induced non-shivering thermogenesis, a process particularly important for hibernating animals. The heat production of this tissue is controlled by the autonomic nervous system. The BAT mitochondria are highly specialized for heat production and contain a unique proton conductance pathway that is controlled by a specialized protein, thermogenin, found in the inner mitochondrial membrane. The operation of the pathway is regulated by purine nucleotides,[11,12] which inhibit proton conductance and also levels of specific long chain fatty acids which remove this inhibition.[13] It has been proposed that this tissue, though small in amount, will increase heat production upon stimulation by the autonomic nervous system when excess energy is ingested, and obese individuals may have a defect in either BAT or in its stimulation.[10,14]

Two questions need to be answered: does adult man have metabolically active BAT and, if so, do obese patients have decreased diet-induced thermogenesis?

After an intravenous injection of ephedrine, a sympathomimetic drug, thermographic 'hot spots' are demonstrable between the shoulder blades and at the back of the neck in man. BAT is stimulated by noradrenaline and ephedrine and in animals is found in similar sites. Therefore, the occurrence of these 'hot spots' is presumptive evidence that BAT is present in man.[10] Though it may be present, its metabolic activity and importance have yet to be quantitated (in rats, BAT receives up to 35% of the cardiac output depending upon the metabolic state of the animal).

A second report suggests that there is reduced thermogenesis in human obesity.[15] In this study, the response of the body's resting oxygen consumption to a noradrenaline infusion was taken as a measure of stimulatable thermogenesis. This measure was reduced in a group of obese women compared with normal-weight control women. In women who had previously been obese but who had dieted and maintained their reduced weight for up to two years, this measure was also reduced.

It is therefore possible that a subgroup of patients with obesity may have absent or inactive BAT. This means that correct therapy in this group of patients would be BAT-stimulation with an appropriate sympathomimetic agent. Such drugs are being developed.

'Futile Cycles'

'Whenever there is a critical interconversion of two metabolic intermediates at a rate-limiting step in a metabolic pathway or at a branching point between two pathways, opposing unidirectional enzymatic reactions are often found. These two reactions provide a sensitivity and degree of control far beyond that provided by mass action through the equilibrium across a single bidirectional enzymatic process' (Sir Hans Krebs as quoted by G.F. Cahill[16]). Simply put, this means that control points in metabolic reactions have 2 enzymes which act in opposite directions; being able to alter the rate of either or both at any one time provides sensitive metabolic control. An example is the interconversion between fructose-6-phosphate (F6P) and fructose biphosphate (FBP) in the glycolytic pathway. Two enzymes are involved (see fig. 10.1); phosphofructokinase which catalyses the forward reaction F6P to FBP and fructose 1,6-biphosphatase which catalyses the reverse. These 2 enzymes constitute a substrate or 'futile' cycle,[17] the operation of which utilizes energy.

Two things are important with these cycles – the amount of cycling and the amount of forward movement from the cycle through the metabolic pathway (flux). The same flux can be obtained with vastly different cycling rate (see fig. 10.2). The operation of these cycles improves sensitivity for metabolic change (sensitivity is proportional to the rate of cycling to flux) and also means that the effects of metabolic change or indiscretion or altered energy input are felt for some time after that change has ceased. The effects of exercise or a meal upon metabolism therefore continue for hours to days after the exercise has ceased or the meal finished. This has important consequences for those attempting to lose weight. Exercise is beneficial because in addition to the calories burned during the exercise, an increased rate of cycling continues for quite some time longer, resulting in a further energy (kilojoule) loss.

With each 'turn' of the cycle energy is lost as heat. It is possible that obese individuals have a low rate of cycling. Therefore less energy is lost as heat for the same flux through a metabolic pathway and more energy is available for storage as fat. Obese individuals are in one sense metabolically efficient but at the expense of easier adipose tissue storage and weight gain (also as a consequence the sensitivity of their metabolic processes to change is reduced).

In summary, if the activity of these cycles is less in obese patients (i.e. they are metabolically more efficient) they will have more energy to store and hence gain weight. This hypothesis has proved difficult to investigate but it remains a possible cause of obesity.

ATP'ases

Na/K ATP'ase is a cell membrane enzyme which helps maintain the intracellular sodium (Na+) concentration. Its activity is essential to the integrity of the cell and it is important in assisting many cellular processes. It is found in all the cells of the body. It is difficult to quantitate the total contribution of the activity of this enzyme to the body's basal energy requirements, but various estimates have been made and these vary between 15% and 80% of the total daily basal energy requirements. Whatever the actual level of the contribution, the activity of this enzyme is significant.

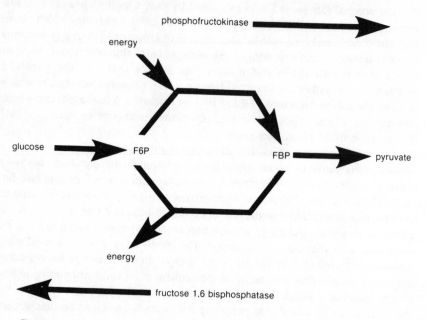

Fig. 10.1 A substrate cycle. Adapted from Newsholme[17].

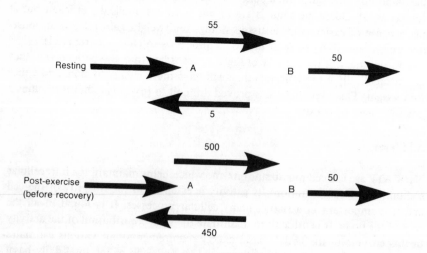

Fig. 10.2 Metabolic flux. Numbers represent 'molecules' passing through pathway. Adapted from Newsholme[17].

A low basal activity of the enzyme might predispose to obesity by its effect upon daily energy requirements and a low activity of this enzyme in the red blood cells of obese patients has been reported.[18] Other workers have failed to find a reduction in activity and in fact reported an increase.[19] The difference in results may be due to technical and assay difficulties. A recent report has suggested there are differences in ATP'ase activity,[20] but these differences are due to ethnic origin (the activity is low in Jewish populations) rather than just to obesity.

The question of activity has to be resolved, but a low level of enzyme activity with a reduction in basal energy requirements would predispose to obesity.

Research continues in these 3 main areas. Though increases in intake will cause obesity, variations in the ability to deal with the energy intake may predispose to and perpetuate obesity and in particular may give an explanation of the wide variation in energy intake reported amongst obese patients. To maintain an increased body weight in normal individuals an increased energy intake is required[21] whilst not all obese patients have a high kilojoule intake.[22]

Secondary Metabolic Changes in Obesity

There are several metabolic changes found in association with the obese state, and there is still debate whether these are the cause of or consequent upon obesity.

Insulin resistance is found in obesity and its most obvious manifestation is hyperinsulinaemia. Such resistance may occur at the cell surface (with changes in receptor number and affinity) or within the cell itself (with changes in enzyme activity).[23] In adipocytes from obese women, insulin receptor number is reduced and glucose transport and oxidation, upon insulin stimulation, are also decreased. A low kilojoule diet for 10 days restores insulin receptor binding and glucose transport to normal, but glucose oxidation remains low.[24] The changes in intracellular enzyme activity are therefore quite long-lasting and by virtue of their existence may predispose to further obesity by preventing glucose oxidation and permitting fat synthesis. In experimental obesity syndromes in animals, such enzyme changes develop early in the course of obesity and appear to be dependent upon the presence of fatty acids for oxidation, which in turn may be dependent upon a critical body adipose tissue mass.[25,26]

It is interesting to note that elevated insulin levels as described in obesity are sufficient to depress thermogenesis following food ingestion.[27]

Endocrine Causes

Though a 'glandular problem' is the major excuse for the occurrence of obesity, in reality, very few obese patients have an underlying hormonal disorder.

The relationship of Type II Diabetes Mellitus to obesity deserves some comment. Hyperinsulinaemia is present in both diabetes and obesity. It is thought to be an expression of the resistance of peripheral tissues to the action of insulin, and is caused by obesity. Currently, it is not clear whether the diabetes which supervenes in obese people (Type II) is due to pancreatic B cell disorders or whether it is consequent upon peripheral resistance. It is possible that peripheral cellular changes may predispose to both obesity and diabetes. Diabetic patients (especially those with Type II) often gain weight when insulin therapy or therapy with oral hypoglycaemics is instigated. These patients have increased insulin-stimulated fat deposition and decreased glucose loss in the urine.

Simple obesity and Cushing's syndrome have many clinical features in common, including general appearance and increased blood levels of steroids (though in obese patients these are easily suppressible by oral dexamethasone). Iatrogenic Cushing's syndrome is far more common than the spontaneous syndrome. The exact mechanism of weight gain is unclear. Changes in food intake do occur with increased steroid levels and it is possible that raised steroid levels lower BMR as well as producing insulin resistance.

In acromegaly there is a general increase in the size of body tissues produced by the high circulating growth hormone levels. In addition these patients may have diabetes.

Hypothyroidism is an unusual cause of obesity. In this disorder some of the overweight is due to the accumulation of fluid in tissues (myxoedema). Triiodothyronine levels respond quickly to changes in energy intake but there is little evidence to suggest that obese patients differ from normal in their thyroid hormone responses.

Sex hormones obviously affect weight and fat distribution as women have a greater body fat content than men, and women do gain weight during pregnancy. Some of this weight is attributable to increased food intake, but hormonal changes may also induce metabolic rate changes. The hyperprolactinaemia of pregnancy probably contributes to this weight gain as patients with raised prolactin alone may be mildly overweight, and on treatment of their high prolactin they will lose weight. After pregnancy the excess body fat should be lost during lactation. Both hypogonadal males and ovariectomized females tend to gain weight. However, a purely endocrine cause for obesity is rare.

Summary

A consideration of the endocrine and metabolic derangements in or caused by obesity leads to logical therapy. Food intake should be watched, remembering that there may be individual variations in basal requirements and the ability to deal with ingested energy. The reasons for excess intake should be pursued and appropriately treated. Energy expenditure should be increased, remembering that altered exercise patterns may produce obesity and that an individual's ability to deal with energy intake may differ.

Logical drug therapy is being developed, and appetite suppressants may have a place in therapy. To achieve weight loss it is obvious that a lasting lifestyle change must be effected by the patient. Such a change must embrace nutritional habits, exercise and any psychological causes for obesity.

References

1. Black, Sir D. (Chairman): Obesity – A report of the Royal College of Physicians. *Journal of the Royal College of Physicians of London* 17: 5-65 (1983).
2. Society of Actuaries: *Build Study 1979* (Association of Life Insurance Medical Directors of America, 1979).
3. Bray, G.A.: The energetics of obesity. *Medicine Science Sport & Exercise* 15: 32-40 (1983).
4. Apfelbaum, M., Bostarron, J. and Lucatis, D.: Effect of calorie restriction and excessive calorie intake on energy expenditure. *American Journal of Clinical Nutrition* 24: 1405-9 (1971).
5. Wilkin, T.J., Choquet, R.C., Schmouker, Y., Rouquette, N., Baldet, L. and Vannereau, D.: Maximum calorie (sub-threshold) dieting of the obese and its hormonal response *Acta Endocrinologica* 103: 184-7 (1983).
6. Miller, D.S. and Parsonage, S.: Resistance to slimming: adaptation or illusion? *Lancet* 1: 773-5 (1975).
7. Ravussin, E., Burnand, B., Shutz, Y. and Jequier, E.: Twenty-four hour energy expenditure and resting metabolic rate in obese, moderately obese and control subjects. *American Journal of Clinical Nutrition* 35: 566-73 (1982).
8. Jung, R.T. and James, W.P.T.: Is obesity metabolic? *British Journal of Hospital Medicine* 24: 503-9 (1980).
9. Griffiths, M. and Payne, P.R.: Energy expenditure in small children of obese and non-obese parents. *Nature* 260: 698-700 (1976).
10. Nicholls, D.G.: Brown adipose tissue mitochrondria. *Biochimica Biophysica Acta* 549: 1-29 (1979).
11. Himms-Hagen, J., Triandafillou, J. and Gwilliam, C.: Brown adipose tissue of cafeteria fed rats. *American Journal of Physiology* 241: E116-E120 (1981).
12. Rial, E., Poustie, A. and Nicholls, D.G.: *European Journal of Biochemistry* 137: 197-203 (1983).
13. Rothwell, N.J. and Stock, M.J.: A role for brown adipose tissue in diet-induced thermogenesis. *Nature* 281: 31-5 (1979).
14. Brooks, S.L., Rothwell, N.J., Stock, M.J., Goodbody, A.E. and Trayhurn, P.: Increased proton conductance pathway in brown adipose tissue mitochrondria of rats exhibiting diet induced thermogenesis. *Nature* 286: 274-6 (1980).
15. Jung, R.T., Shetty, P.S., James, W.P.T., Barrand, M.A. and Callingham, B.A.: Reduced thermogenesis in Obesity. *Nature* 279: 322-3 (1979).
16. Cahill, G.F.: Metabolic Memory. *New England Journal of Medicine* 302: 396-7 (1980).
17. Newsholme, E.A.: A possible metabolic basis for the control of body weight. *New England Journal of Medicine* 302: 400-4 (1980).
18. De Luise, M., Blackburn, G.L. and Flier, J.S.: Reduced activity of the red-cell sodium-potassium pump in human obesity. *New England Journal of Medicine* 303: 1017-22 (1980).
19. Mir, M.A., Charalambous, B.M., Morgan, K. and Evans, P.J.: Erythrocytes, sodium-potassium ATP'ase and sodium transport in obesity. *New England Journal of Medicine* 305: 1264-8 (1981).

20. Beutler, E., Kuhl, W. and Sacks, P.: Sodium-Potassium ATP'ase activity is influenced by ethnic origin and not by obesity. *New England Journal of Medicine* 309: 756-60 (1983).

21. Sims, E.A.H., Danforth, E., Horton, E.S., Bray, G.A., Glennon, J.A. and Salans, L.B.: Endocrine and metabolic effects of experimental obesity of man. *Recent Progress in Hormone Research* 29: 457-96 (1973).

22. Keen, H., Thomas, B.J., Jarrett, R.J. and Fuller, J.M.: Nutrient intake, adiposity and diabetes. *British Medical Journal* 1: 655-8 (1979).

23. Olefsky, J.M.: Lilly Lecture 1980! Insulin Resistance and Insulin Action. An in vitro and in vivo perspective. *Diabetes* 30: 148-62 (1980).

24. Hjollund, E., Pederson, O., and Sorenson, N.S.: Insulin binding and insulin action in fat cells from obese patients before and after fasting. *Diabetologia* 21: 283 A230 (1981).

25. Kerbey, A.L., Caterson, I.D., Williams, P.F. and Turtle, J.R.: Proportion of active dephosphorylated pyruvate dehydrogenase complex in heart and isolated heart mitochondria is decreased in obese hyperinsulinaemic mice. *Biochemical Journal* 217: 117-21 (1984).

26. Caterson, I.D., Williams, P.F., Kerbey, A.L., Plehwe, W.E. and Turtle, J.R.: The effect of body weight and the fatty acid oxidation inhibitor 2 tetradecylgylcidic acid on pyruvate dehydrogenase complex activity in mouse heart. *Biochemical Journal* 224: 787-91 (1984).

27. Danforth, E.: The role of thyroid hormones and insulin in the regulation of energy metabolism. *American Journal of Clinical Nutrition* 38: 1006-17 (1983).

Chapter XI

Hypnosis, Body Image and Weight Control

Introduction

The desire to be slim and to appear youthful has led many individuals to try everything from hypnosis, to having their jaws wired together, to radical surgery.[1] Some success has been achieved when hypnosis has been used alone although Sheehan, Dolby and McDermott reported that the prognosis is better when hypnosis is used as part of a more general treatment programme.[2] In a review of the literature on the use of hypnosis in the treatment of obesity Mott and Roberts concluded that most reports were anecdotal in nature and gave few details of the specific procedures employed.[3] Moreover, they emphasized the need for well-controlled studies which might tease out the relationship between susceptibility and outcome and help discriminate the most effective hypnotic methods in the treatment of different types of obesity. They did, however, conclude that there was some evidence to suggest that hypnosis was effective in the treatment of obesity.

The programme to be outlined in this chapter, unlike others employing hypnotic procedures, involves a method of weight control which progressively monitors movement toward a more desirable or nominated body percept. Through photographing patients, then videotaping the prints, it is possible to change body proportions on a television monitor and actually show patients how they would look if they were slimmer. Patients are able to set their own weight reduction goals and see how they could actually look at the end of the programme. Moreover, they are able to monitor their progress with a series of visual records. Hypnotic suggestions, as they are typically used in weight reduction programmes, serve to enhance overall motivation and visual imagery techniques employed in trance can be reinforced by actual sensory impressions using the video images to enhance the prospects of success.

Body Image

The concept of body image has included surface, depth and postural pictures of the body as well as the attitudes, emotions and personality reactions of individuals toward their bodies.[4] Bennett attempted to define body image operationally when he claimed it to be the set of phenomena named by individuals when they were asked to describe their bodies, reply to a questionnaire about their bodies or draw pictures of them.[5] It is because of the lack of any precise definition of the concept that it has been variously described as body schemata, postural body, perceived body, body ego and body boundaries[4] as well as body concept[6] and body percept.[7]

One of the most widely quoted definitions of body image is 'the picture of our own body which we form in our mind, that is to say the way in which the body appears to ourselves'.[8] Schilder recognized the important relationship among social, psychological and physiological factors in body image formation and argued that body image had a *conscious* and *unconscious* component.[8] Arnhoff and Damianopoulos suggested that studies of body recognition from pictures were an operational way of measuring those aspects of body image which were available to *consciousness*[9] while Jupp and Collins[10] have used the Secord Homonyms Test[11] to measure *unconscious* concerns with the body image.

Persons with deviant body builds generally make more errors in estimating their bodily appearance than persons with normal physiques. Schonbruch and Schell concluded that both overweight and underweight college students tended to overestimate body size and shape.[12] Similarly, Garner *et al.,* using a distorting photography technique, found that anorectic and obese subjects overestimated body size when compared with normal controls.[13] The findings of Gellert *et al.* further support the evidence for distortion of body image in deviant groups.[7] They found that children with average body builds were more accurate in identifying themselves than children with high body fat ratios.

The Technique

The technique was developed following some research on adolescent body recognition. Collins, Harper and Cassel reported that when adolescents were asked to pick their own photograph from an array of 7 photographs with the heads occluded, they used idiosyncratic blemishes to identify themselves.[14] Collins, using a similar technique, reported similar findings when adolescents were asked to identify specific parts of their bodies.[15]

This led to a search for a technique whereby a range of photographs of the same person, distorted in such a way to produce variations from extreme ectomorphy to extreme endomorphy, could be used. The accuracy of body recognition could then be determined while controlling for specific blemishes, self-perceived irregularities of body form or preoccupations arising from over-critical concerns with body form. It was decided to photograph the subjects and use a video-camera to change the dimensions of the photograph. The image on the monitor was varied to provide a continuum ranging through various somato-types so that the accuracy of body recognition could be studied.

Specifically, the video-apparatus consisted of a Sony CC video-camera with a 12.5-75 zoom lens, set to focus at a standard distance of 908mm. The impulses impulses from the video-camera were fed into 288mm Astor professional monitor. The frame size control was disconnected and an external control, with a 2-metre extension cord, was attached. The control knob was graduated on a linear scale which was derived in relation to the rotation of the original frame size control, using one centimetre square graph paper as a gradicle. Images could be varied in the horizontal plane to give an endomorphic, mesomorphic or ecto-morphic figure without distorting height.

A setting of 100 on the frame size control indicated 100% accuracy, a setting of 50 indicated an underestimation of body size by 50% and a setting of 150 indicated an overestimation by 50% of body size. These settings limited the judgments which could be made. Interpolated between these extremes were the estimates of body size, made by the patients, which could be expressed in terms of per cent overestimates or underestimates of body size.

The Programme

Acceptance into the programme was contingent on a medical screening to establish the physical condition of the patient. Individuals with pathological conditions such as endocrine or metabolic dysfunction, unless controlled, were excluded.

The programme included attendance once a week for a period of 15 weeks for an initial induction session followed by 10 clinical sessions involving intensive counselling interspersed with 4 measurement sessions.

Measurements included height which was taken with the head held and looking straight forward with the lower border of the eye sockets in the same horizontal plane as the external auditory meati. Gentle pressure was applied upwards by placing the hand under the mastoid processes to help the subject stretch. Body weight was measured with the subject wearing underclothes only. Three skinfold measures (triceps, subscapula and supra-iliac) were taken with calipers according to the methods outlined by Tanner[16] and Tanner and Whitehouse.[17] Various bodily girths were taken with an anthropometric tape to ensure constant tension. Wrist girth was measured at a point on the narrowest part of the wrist distal to the styloid process of the ulna. Arm girth was measured at a point midway between the superior aspect of the acromial process and the oleocranon process of the elbow. Chest girth or bust measurement was taken at the level of the papillae. Two abdominal girths were measured: the first just below the rib cage and a second at a point just above the anterior superior iliac spine. Buttocks girth was taken at the point of greatest diameter about the external prominences posterior to the hips. Two measures of the thigh were recorded: one approximately half-way between the greater trochanter and the lateral condyle at a point judged to be of greatest thigh circumference and the second at the same place but around both thighs. Calf girth was measured at a point of maximum circumference about the gastrocnemius and soleus muscles, and ankle girth was taken at the narrowest point superior to the medial and lateral malleoli.

Follow-ups were conducted at 1, 3 and 6 months. Progress was continually monitored during this time, including provision for contact within the intervening period if necessary.

The first contact involved a hypnotic induction using the (HGSHS:A) Harvard Group Scale of Hypnotic Susceptibility, Form A,[18] an explanation of the programme and establishing preferences for individual or group counselling. The second session was a measurement session where anthropometric recordings were taken, photographs taken and body percepts established. Measurement sessions were repeated at the sixth, eleventh and fifteenth contacts, then at the follow-up sessions 1, 3 and 6 months later. The entire programme lasted 54 weeks. Clinical sessions were conducted on the third to fifth, seventh to tenth and twelfth to fourteenth contact. During the follow-up sessions either cognitive counselling or hypnosis was given depending on the patient's disposition.

Results

The data reported here have been gathered from a number of different groups of patients who have entered the programme at different times. Some follow-up data are available and are reported here. More will be analysed and made ready for publication in the course of the coming year.

Weight Loss

The mean initial weight of the first 100 patients to complete the programme was 82.89kg (SD = 15.02). At the end of the programme it was 74.56kg (SD = 13.75), which represents a decrease of 10.04%. This decrease was maintained when they were weighed 4 months after the completion of the programme ($\bar{X}$ = 74.41kg, SD = 14.15). At this stage weight reduction was 10.23%. Six months later, that is 10 months after the completion of the programme, their mean weight was 74.01kg (SD = 15.85), which represents a decrease of 10.71%.

Anthropometric Recordings

In a study of 43 females between the ages of 19 and 66 years the mean weight loss over 15 weeks was 7.42kg (SD = 3.98). This represented a 9.27% reduction in body weight. Significant reductions at the 0.01 level were found in all anthropometric recordings. In terms of per cent change, the greatest reductions were found for subscapular measures (14.5), triceps (12.7), abdomen I (11.2), thigh (8.2) and buttocks (7.1). A factor analytic study revealed that 5 factors accounted for 93% of the variance. These were a general weight loss factor (44%), a torso factor (22%), a limb factor (11%), a subcutaneous fat factor (9%) and a thigh girth factor (7%).

These findings enabled refinements to be made in the number of anthropometric recordings worth taking. Besides weight, limb circumference at the arm, thigh and calf should be taken together with a skinfold measure and the traditional truncal measures of bust, abdomen and buttocks. Measures on these variables seemed to account for most of the variance in the factor analysis. Weight loss is not the complete answer in any programme using exercise to affect the enzymatic processes involved in the laying down of fatty deposits. Besides helping to burn energy and use up unnecessary kilojoules, a redistribution of the mass of adipose tissue, muscle and lean tissue takes place which is not reflected in simple weight reduction. Limb and truncal measures help to monitor somatotype change as does a skinfold measure for subcutaneous tissue, perhaps in the tricep area.

Measures of height, symphysis height, finger tip span, body surface area (calculated using the Du Bois-Meeh formula reported by Consolazio, Johnson and Pecora,[19]) and linearity index[20] were recorded to see if lengths of limbs and somatotype had any effect on weight reduction. A significant reduction in body surface area ($\bar{X}$ diff = 0.08m^2, SD = 0.04m^2) and a mean increase in linearity ($\bar{X}$ diff = 0.38, SD = 0.20) were found. The changes in these measures were significant at the 0.001 level. Such changes are to be expected during weight loss. However, the length of limbs bore no significant relationship to weight loss.

Body Recognition and Concern

The accuracy of body recognition was studied using a group of 68 females. A number of interesting results arose from this study. Those patients who dropped out of the programme saw themselves as 26% larger than they actually were. The average age of drop-outs was also younger (35.4 years) than of those who completed the programme (42.4 years). The latter group saw themselves as 19% larger than they actually were when they began the programme and this reduced to 12% by the end of 15 weeks. That is, the error in their body percepts had been reduced considerably.

Before treatment began patients set a goal for themselves (goal photograph) which averaged 8.5% reduction in body contours. The ideal figure that they wished they had (optative photograph) was 17% less than their objective somatotype. By the end of the programme they set a new goal of 21.2% less than their original somatotype and a new optative figure which was not significantly different from this goal; that is, 21.9% reduction. One final piece of information which is of interest is that when the median weight (82.4kg) was used to divide the patients into an obese and a more obese group at the beginning of the programme, the more obese patients considered themselves to be 24% larger than they actually were and the less obese group saw themselves as 19% larger. These findings are consistent with the distortions in body image in deviant groups reported by other workers.[7,12,13] A more elaborate discussion of these results is found in Collins et al.[21]

The Secord Homonym Test[11] was administered to a control group of 74 relatives of students attending a large metropolitan university and a group of 33 obese patients. Prior to the programme the mean score for the obese group was 9.39 (SD = 3.72) which showed significantly more unconscious concern for the body and its functioning than the control group's mean score of 6.29 (SD = 2.61). Retesting after 15 weeks showed the control group's mean concern had not changed significantly, 6.28 (SD = 2.89), whereas the obese group's concern following treatment had dropped to a mean of 6.94 (SD = 2.79) which was now not significantly different from the control group.[22]

A Control Group

A control group of patients was studied to test for the Hawthorne effect[23] or any incentive that may have ensued simply because a patient was enrolled in a weight reduction programme. These patients were inducted into the programme, measured and then informed that actual weight reduction therapy would commence in a further 13 weeks. Before starting therapy measurements were recorded again.

Instead of responding to the incentive of being enrolled in a programme the reverse effect was found in these patients. Weight increased by an average of 0.5kg. Chest circumference and limb circumferences increased by 0.93cm and 0.44cm respectively and skinfold measures increased by 0.16cm. All of these increases were significant at the 0.01 level.

It was as if patients had concluded: 'I am going on a diet shortly so I will make the most of it before my intake is restricted'.

Personality Variables

In the past obese people have been considered to be either jolly, happy and rolypoly or frustrated and unhappy. In the latter case the obesity was often interpreted as the result of frustration. More recently it has been considered that much of the unhappiness associated with obesity may be the result of this condition rather than the cause.

A group of 43 patients were tested before and after treatment for neuroticism and submission using the Neuroticism Scale Questionnaire,[24] for depression using the Minnesota Multiphasic Personality Inventory[25] and for self-esteem using the Personality Research Form.[26] It must be remembered that during hypnosis ego-enhancing suggestions were given. For example, it was suggested that the patients would become more energetic, more vivacious, more vital, happier and more exhuberant. Feelings of well-being, an increase in muscle tone, more efficient circulatory and respiratory systems and a healthier outlook on life were suggested would accompany and be the result of daily exercise.

Following therapy patients' scores reflected significantly less neuroticism ($p < 0.05$), less submission ($p < 0.01$) and less depression ($p < 0.05$). However, no significant change was found in the measures of self-esteem. One other significant change, which was interesting as no specific suggestions relating to it were given and which may be interpreted as reflecting an ease in tension, was a reduction in blood pressure. Systolic readings dropped from 17.2kPa (129mm Hg) before treatment to 16.4kPa (123mm Hg) after treatment ($p < 0.01$) and diastolic from 11.1 to 10.5kPa (83 to 79mm Hg) ($p < 0.05$).

Hypnotic Treatment Effects

An obvious question relates to whether hypnosis as a treatment strategy is more effective with more susceptible patients. The first 100 patients were categorized as low (0-3), medium (4-7) or highly susceptible (8-12) on the HGSHS:A.[18] No significant differences were found in the per cent weight loss among the groups ($F(2,99) = 0.50$, $p = 0.60$).

When the mean initial weight of the low (83.16kg), medium (81.67kg) and highly (83.74kg) susceptible patients was used as a covariate in a repeated measures design over the therapeutic and follow-up sessions, no significance could be attached to the effects of the initial weights of the patients ($F(2,194) = 0.43$, $p = 0.65$). Indeed, no correlation at all was found between hypnotic susceptibility and weight loss when a Peason product-moment correlation coefficient was obtained ($r = 0.00$). As yet a non-hypnosis, non-suggestion control group has not been run to isolate the effects of suggestion.

Being interested in the concept of hypnosis and its measurement as well as its use as a therapeutic technique, the research team administered the HGSHS:A to a group of 29 patients. They were then asked to give a subjective impression of trance depth immediately after induction. An 11-point scale, ranging from 0 to 10, where 0 indicated no trance at all and 10 the deepest trance they could imagine, was used. A correlation of 0.79 (p < 0.001) was found between the HGSHS:A and this scale, indicating the use of a hypnotic barometer in a clinical setting may have some use as a quick indicant of trance depth. When this was replicated on a further group of 81 patients a correlation of 0.70 (p < 0.001) was found.

One interesting treatment effect resulted from different information being given to patients about their trance behaviour. One group was given no information at all. Following therapy no mention was made to this control group about their imagery, how they felt in trance or how deeply they thought they had entered the trance state. A second group was asked to make a judgment on an 11-point scale ranging from 0 for no trance at all to 10, the deepest trance they could imagine. This group was called the subjective impression group. A third group was always led to believe that its members had entered a moderate trance no matter how deep they appeared to go. They were told after each induction 'You appeared to be in a moderate trance today', 'You seemed to have achieved a medium depth ...', 'You responded moderately well to suggestions today', or 'You seemed to be in the middle range of hypnotic depth...'. This group was called the moderate trance group. The final group was called the Challenge group. During the course of each induction they were given ideomotor, challenge and dissociative items. For example, different ideomotor items on various days may have comprised arm levitation, straightening of the arm, or bending the elbow; challenge items may have included the inability to open the eyes, or to bend the arm or to pull the hands apart; and dissociative items may have included hearing a fly buzzing about the face, listening to the beats of music or feeling the skin being touched by a hot instrument.

The first group which was given no information whatsoever lost significantly less weight than the other 3 groups. While this result is only speculative at present and it needs replicating it does indicate that for hypnosis to be effective as an adjuvant to treatment patients should be given some indication that they had entered the trance state. Clarke and Jackson[27] stress that patients are treated in hypnosis not by hypnosis and while concurring with this statement it might be appropriate to add 'when the assumptive state of hypnosis is reinforced by the therapist.'

Most research on hypnotherapy comes from case studies usually performed by a single therapist using a particular treatment strategy. The influence of the sex of the therapist and the type of hypnotic setting has received little attention. Our research team was interested in group versus individual therapy. If the sex of the therapist or the individual setting were to be an influence in hypnotherapy one might expect its presence within the area of weight control where a latent erotic level of interaction between therapist and patient is present through the preoccupation with making the body more attractive. Meares claimed that while the therapist-patient relationship was not an overtly erotic relationship, it probably had primitive erotic elements.[28]

A group of 44 obese females were assigned at random to either a male or a female therapist and at the same time to either group (groups up to 5) or individual therapy. The mean weight loss for the patients treated by female therapists was 7.28kg which represented 9.10% of their body weight. The weight loss of patients treated by male therapists was 7.32kg representing 9.14% of body weight. When group versus individual therapy was studied the patients undergoing group therapy lost 8.24kg representing 10.3% weight loss while the patients treated individually lost 7.2kg representing 9.0% of their original weight. None of these differences were significant and it was concluded that for female patients it is equally effective to work individually or in groups or with male or female therapists.

Discussion

The results reported come from an on-going research programme. They are incomplete and in some respects inconclusive as not all treatment effects have been isolated.

Theories of obesity abound. Biologically based theories include being programmed to eat more,[29] a biological set point, [29] thermogenesis, [30] and dependence on the number of fat cells.[31] Environmentally based theories include the externality hypothesis, [32] the inability to stop eating because of response tendencies or the faulty brake theory, [33] parental influences, [34] our activity levels [35] and maladaptive eating habits.[36]

No single theory can adequately account for obesity. Explanations which include everything tell us nothing, but do indicate a multifaceted approach may be necessary. While the results of traditional medical treatments have been discouraging, behaviour therapy techniques have achieved a modicum of success. The technique outlined above employs traditional hypnotherapeutic techniques, behaviour modification, exercise and diet, ego-enhancing suggestions and a visual goal. Our results suggest that through this blend a certain success can be achieved.

Schachter and Rodin claimed: 'Of all human frailties obesity is the most perverse. The penalties are so severe, the gratifications so limited and the remedy so simple that obesity should be the most trivial of aberrations to correct. Yet it is among the most recalcitrant. Almost any fat person can lose weight, few can keep it off.'[37] As mentioned earlier it was once thought that obese people were unhappy and that their obesity was the result of this unhappiness. From the vast numbers seeking help, it does appear that the unhappiness is the consequence of the obesity and not the cause. It is often the stigma attached to obesity that motivates them to seek help. After therapy the results show patients to be less neurotic, less submissive and less depressed.

Most of the patients are women: approximately 95% of those who have enrolled in the programme. Women are more concerned about their figures than men[38] and since the image of the beautiful woman is thin, most of them wish to lose weight. This has been referred to as the 'what is beautiful is good syndrome'.[39] The studies reported here clearly substantiate the claims that people with deviant body builds overestimate their size when compared to normal controls.[12,13] After therapy their body images were closer to the objective dimensions.

Silverstone and Solomon reported that obese individuals have diminished self-esteem, a lack of worth and are constantly preoccupied with their bodies.[40] The present findings indicated an unconscious concern with their bodies which was remedied by therapy. The counselling included ego-enhancing suggestions and suggestions relating to feelings of well being, becoming more energetic, more vivacious, more vital, becoming healthier, happier and more exuberant, and noticing an increase in muscle tone as well as more efficient circulatory and respiratory systems. More positive perceptions, thoughts, feelings and actions relating to the body probably parallel suggestions and an actual increase in muscle tone with more efficient circulatory and respiratory systems as the change takes place in their somatotypes. These changes are probably then reflected in a diminished unconscious concern.

It is interesting to note that the drop-outs from the programme saw themselves as subjectively larger than those who completed the programme. An explanation for dropping-out could lie in the more unrealistic and more negative stereotypes of their body builds. By exaggerating their obesity they may perceive remediation as hopeless or they may have had unrealistic expectations of magical weight loss which was incompatible with our emphasis on a slow modification of life style. The incapacity to represent the body accurately could be an index of general neuroticism and it could be argued dynamically that the misrepresentation reflects an unconscious need to maintain the symptom.

Finally, the results indicate that susceptibility to hypnosis is not related to weight loss. Cooke and Van Vogt noted that neither medium nor deep trance was necessary to obtain definite benefits from hypnotic suggestions and that even in hypnoidal states patients are more responsive to suggestions than normally.[41] Relaxation therapy was included as part of the hypnotic induction and while susceptibility to suggestions was not found to be a significant factor it is interesting to note that giving information to patients about trance behaviour seemed to be important.

In summary, the therapy seems to be effective over a 15-week period. Patients become more realistic about their subjective body image, they are less concerned about their bodies, less neurotic, less submissive and less depressed. Follow-up studies indicate lasting effects, group therapy is effective and susceptibility to hypnosis is not related to weight loss.

References

1. Hankins, N.E. and Hopkins, A.L.: Locus of control and weight loss in joiners and non-joiners of weight reduction organisations. *Psychological Reports* 43: 11-14 (1978).
2. Sheehan, P.W., Dolby, R.M. and McDermott, D.: Report on hypnotherapeutic techniques and their function. *Australian Psychologist* 10: 213-23 (1975).
3. Mott, R. and Roberts, J.: Obesity and hypnosis: a review of the literature. *American Journal of Clinical Hypnosis* 22: 3-7 (1979).
4. Kolb, L.: Disturbances of body image; in S. Arieti (Ed.) *American Handbook in Psychiatry* (Basic Books, New York 1959).
5. Bennett, D.: The body concept. *Journal of Mental Science* 106: 56-75 (1960).
6. Zion, L.: Body concept as it relates to self concept. *Research Quarterly* 36: 490-5 (1965).
7. Gellert, E., Girgus, J. and Cohen, J.: Children's awareness of their bodily appearance: a developmental study of factors associated with the body percept. *Genetic Psychology Monographs* 84: 109-74 (1971).
8. Schilder, P.: *The Image and Appearance of the Human Body* p.104 (Kegan Paul, London 1935).
9. Arnhoff, F. and Damianopoulos, E.: Self-body recognition: an empirical approach to the body image. *Merrill-Palmer Quarterly* 8: 143-8 (1962).
10. Jupp, J.J. and Collins, J.K.: Instruments for the measurement of unconscious and conscious aspects of body image. *Australian Journal of Clinical and Experimental Hypnosis* 11: 89-100 (1983).
11. Secord, P.F.: Objectivication of word association procedures by the use of homonyms: a measure of body cathexis. *Journal of Personality* 21: 479-95 (1953).
12. Schonbruch, S.S. and Schell, R.E.: Judgments of body appearance by fat and skinny male college students. *Perceptual and Motor Skills* 24: 999-1002 (1967).
13. Garner, D.M., Garfinkel, P.E., Stancer, H.C. and Moldofsky, H.: Body image disturbance in anorexia nervosa and obesity. *Psychosomatic Medicine* 38: 327-36 (1976).
14. Collins, J.K., Harper, J.F. and Cassel, A.J.: Self-body recognition in late adolescence. *Australian Psychologist* 11: 153-7 (1976).
15. Collins, J.K.: Self-recognition of the body and its parts during late adolescence. *Journal of Youth and Adolescence* 10: 243-54 (1981).
16. Tanner, J.M.: *Growth at Adolescence* (Blackwell Scientific Publications, London 1962).
17. Tanner, J.M. and Whitehouse, R.H.: Standards for subcutaneous fat in British children. *British Medical Journal* 1: 446-50 (1962).
18. Shor, R.E. and Orne, E.C.: *The Harvard Group Scale of Hypnotic Susceptibility, Form A* (Consulting Psychologists Press, Palo Alto, California 1962).
19. Consolazio, C.F., Johnson, R.E. and Pecora, L.J.: *Physiological Measures of Metabolic Function in Man* (McGraw-Hill, New York 1963).
20. Parnell, R.W.: Simplified somatotypes. *Journal of Psychosomatic Research* 8: 311-15 (1964).
21. Collins, J.K., McCabe, M.P., Jupp, J.J. and Sutton, J.E.: Body percept change in obese females following weight reduction therapy. *Journal of Clinical Psychology* 37: 507-11 (1983).
22. Jupp, J.J., Collins, J.K., McCabe, M.P., Walker, W.L. and Diment, A.D.: Change in unconscious concern with body image following treatment for obesity. *Journal of Personality Assessment* 47: 483-9 (1983).

23. Roethlisberger, F.J. and Dickson, W.J.: *Management and the Worker* (Harvard University Press, Cambridge, Mass. 1939).

24. Cattell, R.B. and Scheier, I.H.: *Neuroticism Scale Questionnaire* (Institute for Personality and Ability Testing, Champaign, Ill. 1961).

25. Hathaway, S.R. and McKinley, J.C.: *Minnesota Multiphasic Personality Inventory: Manual for Administration and Scoring* (Psychological Corporation, New York 1967).

26. Jackson, D.N.: *Personality Research Form Manual* (Research Psychologists Press, Goshen, New York 1967).

27. Clarke, J.C. and Jackson, A.J.: *Hypnosis and Behavior Therapy* (Springer Publishing Co., New York 1983).

28. Meares, A.: *A System of Medical Hypnosis* (Julian Press, New York 1972).

29. Nisbett, R.E.: Hunger, obesity and the ventromedial hypothalamus. *Psychological Review* 79: 433-52 (1972).

30. Rothwell, N.J. and Stock, M.J.: A role for brown adipose tissue in diet-induced thermogenesis. *Nature* 281: 31-5 (1979).

31. Knittle, J.L.: Obesity in childhood: A problem in adipose tissue cellular development. *Journal of Pediatrics* 81: 1048-59 (1972).

32. Schachter, S.: *Emotion, Obesity and Crime* (Academic Press, New York 1971).

33. Singh, D.: Role of response habits and cognitive factors in the determination of behavior of obese humans. *Journal of Personality and Social Psychology* 27: 220-38 (1973).

34. Goldblatt, P.B., Moore, M.E. and Stunkard, A.J.: Social factors in obesity. *Journal of the American Medical Association* 192: 97-100 (1965).

35. Mayer, J.: Inactivity as a major factor in adolescent obesity. *Annals of the New York Academy of Sciences* 131: 502-6 (1965).

36. Brightwell, D.R. and Clancy, J.: Self-training of new eating behavior for weight reduction. *Diseases of the Nervous System* 37: 85-9 (1976).

37. Schachter, S. and Rodin, J.: *Obese Humans and Rats* (Lawrence Erlbaum, Hillsdale, N.J. 1974).

38. Berscheid, E., Walster, W. and Bournstedt, G.: The happy American body. *Psychology Today* 7: 123 (1973).

39. Dion, K., Berscheid, E. and Walster, W.: What is beautiful is good. *Journal of Personality and Social Psychology* 24: 285-90 (1972).

40. Silverstone, J.T. and Solomon, T.: Psychiatric and somatic factors in the treatment of obesity. *Journal of Psychosomatic Research* 9: 249 (1965).

41. Cooke, C.E. and Van Vogt, A.E.: *The Hypnotism Handbook* (Borden Publishing Co., Alhambra, Calif. 1965).

Chapter XII

The Significance to Behavioural Therapies of Radical Treatments for Massive Obesity

This chapter describes the behaviour of massively obese patients before and after radical treatments such as bypass surgery and dental fixation. These forms of intervention produce dramatically different and novel patterns of weight change in the obese compared with conservative treatments such as behaviour modification, and thus can contribute new information relevant to the aetiology of obesity and to improvements in the management of that problem. The study of obesity in the context of radical intervention has been the subject of several reviews.[1-4] To date none of these reviews have considered dental fixation.

The observations reported come from 4 studies carried out by the author with massively obese subjects. Two of these concern English populations who underwent ileojejunostomy procedures; these have been partially reported upon.[5-7] The remaining 2 populations are Australian and have had dental fixation and gastric bypass procedures.

Some 250 patients in all have been investigated. They are all morbidly obese in the sense that they are in excess of 100% over their standard body weight. They are characteristically patients who have had a wide array of treatments which have ultimately failed, who have mutiple physical, psychological and social problems and who, in general terms, appear to have abandoned hope of ever losing weight. The mean weight of our population was 130 kilograms (plus or minus 20 kilograms), their mean age was 35 (plus or minus 15 years) and their mean weight loss was 45 kilograms with a range of 20 to 60 kilograms. All patients were followed for periods of 2 to 3 years. The majority were female.

Bypass procedures involve a major operation and a general anaesthetic. Dental fixation is treatment evolved to enable patients who are massively obese to lose large amounts of weight with a much greater margin of safety than that which characterizes bypass surgery.[9] Whilst it is known that bypass surgery is a very successful technique and has a high degree of patient acceptance it nonetheless carries a small operative and postoperative mortality rate and a degree of morbidity. Dental fixation only requires that the teeth be wired together. However bizarre that may seem it is readily accepted by patients; it is a very safe procedure.[9] Dental fixation generates similar degrees of weight loss as that found in bypass surgery. The problem with this approach is that all but about 20% of patients regain weight steadily over the 2 years following unwiring. Some do this rapidly and some slowly. There is a general trend for a majority of patients to be able to sustain a degree of weight control for 2 to 3 months after unwiring.

This chapter will discuss 5 areas of concern to all those interested in obesity research:

1. eating behaviour;
2. weight losing behaviour;
3. weight maintenance and weight gaining behaviour;
4. compliance and adherence in treatment regimes;
5. body image disturbances.

Under each of these headings I will report briefly on the general observations about massively obese patients and the observations one can make from radical treatments and then attempt to draw some lessons from these observations for the behavioural therapist.

Eating Behaviour

Most studies of the eating behaviour of the mild to moderately obese report a range of deviant patterns.[10-13] Unfortunately there has been very little study of the massively obese.

Aberant patterns of eating described for the obese include:

1. **Addictive eating** – here the obese subject is construed as somebody who is addicted to food, particularly good-tasting foods, who cannot resist the compulsion to eat and when prevented from doing so suffers a considerable dysphoria.

2. **Reactive hyperphagia** –here the obese subject reports that between periods of dieting or reasonable control there is bingeing. This bingeing takes on qualities familar to those who have worked with bulimic patients of more normal weight.[14-17] The term 'reactive' is used because the obese perceive their bingeing as occurring in response to depression, anxiety, frustration, interpersonal difficulties and sometimes simply to boredom.

3. **Counterregulatory eating** –the form of eating here is perhaps not too different from that described in (1) or (2) above. The concept was devised by Herman and Polivy[18] as an extension of Schachter's externality theory and is reviewed by Wardle and Beinart.[19] This describes a population of the obese who appear to be in a state of chronic restraint; they are always preoccupied with food, always aware that they could gain weight and show many of the characteristics which are familiar to us from psychological studies of patients with anorexia nervosa. They are, as a population, quite similar to the 'thin/fat' population described by Bruch.[20] The key issue with this population is that once eating begins, it escalates to marked overeating rather than a return to constraint or a feeling of satiation.

4. **Unconscious eating** – this is a term used to describe the fact that many obese people either deny having eaten or fail to report eating and yet can note that food previously present in the house is now 'missing'. Whatever mechanism one wishes to use to explain this phenomenon it is certainly very common in the massively obese.

5. **Nibbling** – this is a form of eating which is thought to be distinct in pattern from that described for the population of weight disordered patients who demonstrate bingeing or reactive hyperphagia. It describes a population who seem to eat a small amount very frequently, or more or less continuously.

6. **Night starvation and night bingeing** – Stunkard[11] described a rare eating deviancy in the obese whereby good control is exercised during the daytime together with apparent good adjustment. Both of these break down during the night, the patient demonstrating marked nocturnal eating and extreme personal distress and agitation.

The kinds of information that might be very interesting to a behaviour therapist such as long-term predisposing factors to overeating, the immediate stimuli to bingeing, clear descriptions of the pattern of eating, and the affective and cognitive states in the obese during eating are substantially lacking.

Our preliminary analysis of our own massively obese populations shows that more than half of them demonstrate the pattern described as reactive hyperphagia, that nibbling in the continuous manner is common but that the night eating syndrome is quite rare. One of the most common patterns in the massively obese is daytime dieting (or complete fasting) and gorging or bingeing in the evenings. Part of this behaviour could be considered to be similar to the counterregulatory behaviour described by Herman and may be of considerable relevance to the propensity of the massively obese to gain excess fat stores.[21]

All authors who have studied the effects of bypass surgery on eating behaviour have reported:

1. That after operation eating returns to a conventional pattern irrespective of how abnormal it was before operation. The frequency and duration of meals and the amount eaten follows a normal pattern and is of an amount which is sufficient to maintain a stable weight.

2. Addictive eating, which appears to be relatively common in the massively obese, seems to disappear.[1]

3. There is a very obvious reduction in reactive hyperphagia. This may in part relate to the fact that patients generally report that they are more outgoing, more comfortable being assertive in frustrating situations, and in general happier. Thus the stimuli to reactive hyperphagia may be markedly reduced.

In contradistinction to the patients preoperative expectations – that after the operation they will be able to eat heartily and as much as they like of everything that they had denied themselves – and in contradistinction to much of theoretical literature on obesity which currently centres around the notion of a set point hypothesis (which predicts that the obese who lose a lot of weight would show a gross exaggeration of the psychology and biology of starvation and thus would show a great tendency towards excess energy storage), [19,22] the massively obese after operation report a similar sense of hunger and satiety as those who have never had energy balance problems.

The obese are usually characterized as showing a dissociation between the normal physiology of hunger and conscious reports of the wish to eat.[23]

The emergence of a normal psychology and biology of eating in the massively obese after operation is a remarkable finding.

It is so surprising that it has been considered that there must be some major biological resetting of the total regulatory system of organism towards a new set point as a function of the alteration in bowel anatomy and physiology.[4,13]

I would differ a little with reports of Solow,[4] who feels that the results of gastric bypass surgery are more or less identical with those of ileojejunol bypass surgery. Our own observations would be that this is substantially true, but that there are a minority of patients who have gastric bypass surgery who still continue to overeat and who have much smaller degrees of weight loss and retain a tendency to regain weight.

It is interesting that when ileojejunostomy is reversed, weight is gained to premorbid levels quite rapidly. This is associated with reinstitution of eating patterns of the massively obese prior to operation.

Following dental fixation the recommended diet is 3350 kilojoule mixed fluid diet with vitamin and mineral supplementation. In this situation the following observations can be made about the eating behaviour of patients.

1. A minority (10% to 15%) leave the programme prematurely. There is often a sense of considerable urgency about the patient's need to have the wires cut. This appears to relate to their need to eat and the discomfort of deprivation. Some patients who continue in the programme for 3 to 9 months and hence lose 20 to 50 kilograms continue to report craving and note that from time to time they feel an exaggerated need to 'taste something interesting'.

2. Despite having dental fixation, compliance or adherence problems remain for the massively obese. It is common for patients to break their diets, and some

have in fact gained weight despite dental fixation. This breaking of diet tends to occur at times of increasing interpersonal difficulties within the patient's social system or when the individual herself reports going through a period of depression or anxiety. Patients who do break their diets do sometimes report a craving for sweet-tasting foods, which is the behaviour one would expect from the set point hypothesis outlined above.

Nevertheless it is striking that the experience of the dental fixation patients is much more similar to reports of patients with bypass surgery than of patients with long-term dieting programmes.

Most patients report a sense of security whilst wired which can be associated with a degree of euphoria and elation. The majority of patients report no regular desire to eat nor any obvious major sense of hunger. The dysphoria of dieting 'dieting depression' is uncommon.

3. The situation does tend to change shortly before the patient is due for unwiring. Some then report a sense of anxiety about how they will cope once the constraint of wiring is removed, whilst others believe that they have solved the problems of their obesity and that they will not again become fat.

Although the situation of having one's jaws wired is different from that of self-imposed restraint, we nonetheless consider that there were parallels between this situation and some of the classical behavioural strategies known to induce reasonable weight loss in the obese.[24] Dental fixation is obviously a dramatic way of breaking up an eating pattern. It obviously could make patients more conscious of what they eat, where they eat and what stimulates it. One could image that it could become a form of response prevention such as has been used in obsessive-compulsive disorders.

During the course of being wired most patients report a greatly increased awareness of when and how they ate prior to wiring, and of the stimuli that had induced a binge. They also noted the development of alternative strategies for dealing with personal dysphoria and interpersonal difficulties. All of this would normally be a joy to the ear of a good behaviourally oriented therapist.

Whilst acknowledging that there was a greater degree of passivity in the situation of wiring than in the active participation of a patient in response prevention programmes, it nonetheless is somewhat surprising and extremely disappointing to us that weight gain so regularly occurred in populations who have had severe disruptions of eating patterns for 4 to 9 months. Certainly notions such as the extinction of behaviour following the prolonged absence of reinforcements do not appear to apply in this situation.

There was some hint in our data that the more rapid phases of weight gain after unwiring did not begin until some 2 or 3 months had passed. It is possible, but we could not elicit the information historically, that the patient made use of the insights they had gained during the unwiring, but this could not be sustained. It was certainly true that eating patterns and the stimuli for overeating that characterized our population prior to wiring returned in the first year after unwiring and produced considerable weight gain.

It does seem that where a situation can be devised which radically alters eating behaviour over a long period of time, that patients do become much more aware of themselves, the people in their lives and their own personal goals.

Looking at the results of bypass surgery and dental fixation it would be fair to conclude that powerful interventions are necessary to induce permanent and enduring change in eating patterns and in the experience of hunger and satiety in the morbidly obese. The links between eating and the affective and interpersonal life of the massively obese seems only to change when there is a relatively permanent guarantee of not being able to eat. In the absence of such guarantees the only alternative at present is for the 'thinned obese' to adopt a posture of 'constant restraint.'[18]

It may make more sense for a behavioural therapist to concentrate on the skills required to deal with the unpleasantness of constant restraint than for them to try to induce enduring changes in the basic psycho-physiology of the experience. There are patients who apparently can spontaneously arrive at a constant and reasonably comfortable position of lifetime restraint. The price is high but many patients might consider it worthwhile.

Weight Losing Behaviour

To lose 6 kilograms takes 4 weeks of near total starvation. Losing weight is a very slow process. It is probably for this reason that most behavioural programmes last for 8 to 12 weeks and report weight losses of the order of 3 to 5 kilograms.[24]

It is easy to see that a patient who has to lose up to 50 or more kilograms to be considered modestly obese is not usually a realistic prospect for a conservative treatment programme. However, spontaneous weight loss in the massively obese of quite considerable amounts is not unknown, and many therapists have had the occasional experience of helping a massively obese patient lose 40 or 50 kilograms using combinations of therapies such as behaviour therapy, dynamic psychotherapy and family therapy.

It is not clear whether there are any physiological constraints to the amount of weight that can be lost. The animal literature, and to an extent the human literature, appears to demonstrate that there is a certain normalcy in the total energy stores that an obese individual carries and that as one attempts to reduce weight the body mobilizes a range of defences that are aimed at preventing further depletion of lipid stores and promoting weight gain.[22,23]

There are certainly psychosocial obstructions to permanent weight loss. People important to the obese subject are often ambivalent about weight loss and will interfere with the progress of management.[6,24] It is also true that some of the patients, either consciously or unconsciously, fear that if they become thin they may behave in an unacceptable manner.[6] As mentioned earlier the amount of weight loss after bypass surgery is considerable in extent (20 to 60 kilograms) and on the whole rapid over a period of 6 to 7 months before any plateau effects are noted. This is also true of dental fixation, although a general untested impression in our own unit is that the plateau effect emerges somewhat earlier than is the case for bypass surgery. In conservative treatments the plateau effect has been thought to reflect the general resistance of the obese person (for whatever reasons, be they psychological, social, physiological) to further weight loss.[23] The degree of weight loss in radical procedures is so substantial that it must cast some doubt on the notion that resistance to weight loss in a physiological sense plays a decisive part in the more limited weight losing pattern of those who are on a conservative dietary regime. One surmises that the capacity for losing weight is greater than has previously been suggested.[23,26]

It is certainly the case in both bypass surgery and dental fixation that other elements of resistance to change can be observed. Responses of spouses and families are often intense and ambivalent. The patients themselves often do become fearful that they will neglect their families or their children or break up their marriages as their weight begins to get lower. Certainly many are aware of a propensity to more seductive behaviour which sometimes does verge on genuine promiscuity. Some also demonstrate a much lower tolerance of others and are prone to a degree of assertion which the subjects themselves find somewhat unacceptable. A few become psychotic or severely neurotic.

These observations would be consistent with some of the more recent work of the behaviourists who have emphasized the need to combine personal and marital psychotherapy with a behavioural programme.[24] There is also some evidence that the active participation in a programme of a spouse, who is equally contracted to cooperation as the subject, improves weight loss.[27]

In some respects neither the dental fixation nor the bypass patients provide overwhelming support for the biological set point concept. The dental fixation patients, for example, did not frequently report counter-regulatory behaviour or a marked excess of food preoccupation as the degree of weight loss increased.

Weight Maintenance and Weight Gaining Behaviour

All obesity programmes face the problem of patients who successfully lose weight but then fail to be able to maintain their new-found low weight status.[24] This has perhaps been one of the most disappointing aspects of the behavioural programmes which report good weight loss and often continuing weight loss after the cessation of the programme.

It is the failure to regain weight after bypass surgery which is its most unique feature. This allows us some clues as to some of the issues which the obese person might face if they are to maintain lower weights. As noted above, eating behaviour is remarkably altered in bypass patients and this in a manner which appears to require no special cognitive effort. One must presume that this is a central and important component of the patient's new-found capacity for weight control. There are, however, some other important issues which might be important to a management programme of a more conservative nature in the weight maintenance phase of the treatment.

The reports of psychological and social outcome after bypass surgery are, in general, positive. Close inspection shows that many patients, however, go through quite troubling periods in the first year or two following the achievement of more normal weight.[6,7] Perhaps the most common of these are interpersonal problems between husband and wife, or between the obese subject and her children or the obese subject and her family of origin. Considerable problems within marriages have been reported. This author has seen several spouses become psychotic, mainly with paranoid delusions, after weight loss. Major sexual disturbance is common and many marriages have come under severe strain although not many have broken up.

The parents of subjects often make quite hurtful and ambiguous remarks. It is striking that a good number of our bypass patients moved residence after successfully losing weight (and staying that way) and gave as one of their main reasons 'to put a greater distance between them and their parents'. Similarly, the spouse's children, although broadly speaking pleased, are often confused and perplexed by, not only the change in their mother's shape but also the change in her attitudes and social involvement. It is not always easy for an obese person, who has successfully lost a lot of weight, to be tolerant of these unwelcome responses in her day to day life.

In the case of dental fixation the patients report similar interpersonal disturbances and responses to those experienced by bypass surgery patients. This, together with the rise in personal anxiety and depression, which was very common in both groups of subjects for short periods after weight loss, often contributed to a general sense of turmoil and in some cases chaos.

Another issue which is perhaps not well appreciated is that an obese patient who has lost 60 to 70 kilograms and finds herself relatively thin and relatively attractive may have major problems with her sense of identity. Many of our patients had not been as thin as they were after the operation or after dental fixation for some 20 years – often since the beginning of adolescence. One can presume that their commonly expressed feelings of uncertainty about 'who they were' and the long period of time it took for them to 'recognize themselves in a mirror without surprise' related to this struggle to come to terms with their new identity.

These personal and interpersonal issues are precisely of a kind which the obese person associates with breaking diets in the weight-losing phase of conservative treatments and with bingeing behaviour (reactive hyperphagia) outside of a treatment setting. In the case of dental fixation, the patients, after unwiring, are also presumably faced with the exaggerated biological propensity to gain weight.

In the case of bypass surgery these issues wax and wane over several years; in dental fixation patients a general impression is that the patients can 'hold out' for a few months and then find the struggle too great.

I think these observations emphasize the length of time that a therapist may need to consider putting into the maintenance phase of therapy. This phase should be seen as a separate challenge. It is quite likely that many patients, and not just the massively obese, may take several years to readjust to a lower weight and to gain sufficient strategies and sufficient competence to combat the general tendency to regain weight.

These observations also suggest that the therapist may need to concentrate on providing time for ventilation of distress and for counselling with marital couples or families as well as endeavouring to help the patient find new coping strategies.

I am not suggesting here that the therapist necessarily needs to see the patient at very regular intervals for 2 to 3 years. I suspect that an intense short programme of perhaps 10 weeks after goal weight is achieved may be enough to give the patient a good start. After that time there may need to be a regular programme of follow-up.

The patient also needs to feel that if things are getting out of hand they can contact the therapist. I should mention here that the obese person in the maintenance phase of therapy is much more likely to turn up for appointments or contact you spontaneously if she is doing well than if she is doing badly. A lot of time needs to be put into encouraging the patient to come at times of 'negative progress'.

Compliance and Adherence Issues

A failure to adhere to a mutually agreed upon programme and dropping out is a major issue for all obesity management regimes.[28] This is often attributed to a lack of motivation if one is feeling puritanical or to the fact that the task is very difficult if one is not.

At a behavioural level it is common for obese people to attribute dropping out to their failure to lose weight because they have been eating inappropriately; they often feel ashamed or as if 'they have let the therapist down'.

These variables are not of substantial practical significance in bypass surgery or dental fixation (at least whilst the patient is wired). Indeed, one of the reasons that the procedures were advanced in the first place was because they circumvented compliance problems.

However, the same general behaviour permeates radical programmes. Both bypass surgery and dental fixation patients require regular clinical follow-up for health and research purposes. All of our patients are aware of this need and know that it is medically important. In our programmes they contract, prior to the beginning of their treatment, to be followed up at 6-weekly intervals for 2 years.

An untested, but strong, impression is that non-adherence and dropping out is a much bigger problem in the massively obese than in the mild to moderately obese. Certainly, historically, they are characterized by having sought innumerable treatments which have been shortlived.[6]

In our own treatment programmes we have found that adherence to the follow-up routine is so poor that we have routinely employed a person whose sole task is to keep contact with the patients, to phone to remind them of appointments or to chase them up when they fail to attend.

Even so, less than a third of our dental fixation patients attended more than 80% of their appointments.

In a behaviour modification study of 35 massively obese patients which aimed at weekly sessions for 20 weeks, and were deliberately arranged for the convenience of the patient and also were not conducted in a hospital setting, 55% attended less than 4 sessions. We have had a similar experience with a double-blind trial of medication which was intended to last for a minimum of 6 months. Here, 50% of our subjects had dropped out of the programme in the first 4 weeks.

To what should such poor adherence be attributed?

Our preliminary analysis of failure to attend hospital clinic appointments shows that the behaviour is not related to age, physical disability, whether the patient has private transport or not, the length of time it takes to get to hospital, the usual length of waiting to see the doctor, marital status or whether or not the patient has young children. These are all demographic factors which have been related to poor compliance in other management programmes.[29]

This suggests to us that poor compliance is one example of an enduring personality characteristic of the obese. It is possible that it reflects the social avoidance behaviour associated with, for example, their body image disturbance. It is not related, as far as we can see, to the generally high levels of neuroticism and psychiatric symptomatology which characterize the massively obese seeking help from hospitals;[13] indeed, high levels of neuroticism and anxiety may predict better compliance – the fearful, highly aroused patient is more motivated to seek help. It may be related to the personality characteristic of 'ineffectualness' described by Bruch which so pervades the obese person's lifestyle.[20]

I am suggesting here that dropping out and the failure to adhere to pro-grammes are behaviours which require much closer analysis from behaviourists and a putting aside of previously held assumptions. It is fairly obvious that a client who seeks help must first be able to make regular contact with the ther-apist.

Body Image Issues

One of the few issues that marks the psychological experiences of the obese out from other psychobiological disorders is the presence of body image disturb-ances. Here the patient has a pronounced sense of self-loathing, which behav-iourally is associated with considerable social avoidance behaviour.[13,30] The massively obese are also prone to overestimate their actual body size.[31]

The avoidance behaviours associated with body image disturbance lead to seclusiveness and isolation, which are experienced by the massively obese as frustrating and a source of despair. This, in turn, leads to excessive eating. Such avoidance of course also leads to reduced physical activity which could add its own propensity to weight gain.

Body image disturbance is common in the obese and present in the majority of the massively obese. It appears most often in those who have been obese in adolescence – developmentally the time of identity formation.[30] It has usually been considered to be particularly resistant to change. The only treatment to date which has produced significant change in body image disturbance is psy-choanalysis,[32] and here the change was also associated with substantial weight loss, apparently as a function of treatment, although losing weight had not been an objective of the analysis.

Following bypass surgery the ramifications of body image disturbance are remarkably decreased and social avoidance behaviour diminishes.

Following dental fixation the same changes are seen but are reversed if weight gain occurs. This contrast (with bypass surgery) suggests that the propensity to self-loathing is an abiding characteristic of the obese, but that it can be overrid-den by changed circumstances. It should be noted that there are always some obese people who continue to show body image disturbances and social avoid-ance behaviour no matter how much weight is lost. Some patients are endlessly preoccupied with a 'fold of skin' or 'stretch marks' to a degree which is obviously pathological.

These observations suggest that a behaviourist who chose to ignore weight loss (relatively speaking) as a principal goal of therapy and instead concentrated on: a) the capacity of the massively obese to overcome their sense of helplessness: b) to confront their avoidance behaviour, and c) to bolster their ability to be assertive, might do much to improve the quality of the massively obese patient's life, even if no weight change occurred. All of these treatment objectives are well within the range of good behaviour therapy. In any event one could easily imagine that the coping devices learnt would counteract the sequelae of body image disturbance, and so some weight loss might occur, or at least some ability to control weight rise.

Summary

The changes in behaviour and attitudes observed in the massively obese following bypass surgery and dental fixation are striking and may tell us something fundamental about the nature of obesity and its management.

There are professional and clinical realities which in the past have mitigated against adequate consideration of the findings of radical treatments by behaviourists.

The ideas presented here are not exhaustive – there are many other issues which could have been considered – but the areas chosen are probably the most important for those interested in weight disorder.

My own present conclusions are:

1. That for many overweight people who wish to be permanently thinner; the price paid in the absence of a radical treatment is the development of a 'thin/ fat' psychology and biology. This leaves the person in a state characterized by a preoccupation with food, a preoccupation with the fear of loss of control and also predisposed to abnormal eating such as hyperphagia. Many of these patients also suffer from a degree of overarousal and dysphoria. The fact that a considerable number of modestly obese and normal weight individuals have learnt to live reasonably comfortable lives, despite this experience, suggests that behaviourists might concentrate attention on helping patients to achieve and maintain such a posture.

2. That obstruction to weight loss and maintenance of lower weights is not purely physiological, although that is important. Much more weight could potentially be lost by most obese people than is usually acknowledged.

3. That the weight maintenance phase of treatment requires strategies and much more attention than has previously been considered.

4. That the length of time of treatment needs to be long and more attention needs to be paid to the interpersonal and social aspects of the person's world, and

5. That social avoidance behaviour in the massively obese, secondary to body image disturbance, is a source of a vicious circle, resulting in an escalation of weight. This area would seem to be a very rich source of interest to the behaviourists since so much of it centres around avoidance behaviour, helplessness, low self-esteem and problems in self-assertion.

Finally, I have noted a trend for behaviourists to leave the field of obesity – perhaps discouraged by the complex problems that it presents. The thrust of this chapter is that there is much that the behaviour therapist can do. The aims and objectives of treatment need some rethinking.

References

1. Kalucy, R.S.: Ileo-jejunostomy and its significance for obesity research. *Proceedings of the 1977 Geigy Psychiatric Symposium* – 'Psychiatry in the General Hospital' pp. 89-93.
2. Bray, G.A.: Jejunoileal bypass, jaw wiring and vagotomy for massive obesity; in Stunkard (Ed.) *Obesity*, pp. 369-87 (W.B. Saunders Co, Philadelphia 1980).
3. Halmi, K.: Gastric bypass for massive obesity; in Stunkard (Ed.) *Obesity*, pp. 388-94 (W.B. Saunders & Co., Philadelphia 1980).
4. Solow, C.: Surgical treatment of obesity; in Goodstein (Ed.) *Eating and Weight Disorders. Advances in Treatment and Research*, pp. 32-90 (Springer Publishing Co., New York 1983).
5. Gazet, J-C., Pilkington, T.R.E., Kalucy, R.S., Crisp, A.H., and Day, S.: Treatment of gross obesity by jejunal bypass. *British Medical Journal* 691: 311-14 (1974).
6. Kalucy, R.S., and Crisp, A.H.: Some psychological and social implications of massive obesity. A study of some psychosocial accompaniments of major fat loss occurring without dietary restriction in massively obese patients. *Journal of Psychosomatic Research* 18: 465-73 (1974).
7. Crisp, A.H., Kalucy, R.S., Pilkington, T.R.E., and Gazet, J-C.: Some psychosocial consequences of ileojejunal bypass surgery. *American Journal of Clinical Nutrition* January, 109-20 (1977).
8. Rogers, S., Burnet, R., Goss, A., Philips, P.J., Goldney, R., Kimbre, C., Thomas, D.W., Harding, P.E., and Wise, P.H.: Jaw wiring in the treatment of obesity. *Lancet* 1: 1221-3 (1977).
9. Goss, A.N.: Management of patients with jaws wired for obesity. *British Dental Journal*, 146(11): 339-42 (1979).
10. Hamburger, W.W.: Emotional aspects of obesity. *Medical Clinics of North America* 35: 483-99 (1951).
11. Stunkard, A.J.: Eating patterns and obesity. *Psychiatric Quarterly*, 33: 284-95 (1959).
12. Bruch, H.: Psychological aspects of overeating and obesity. *Psychosomatics*, 5: 268-74 (1964).
13. Kalucy, R.S.: Obesity: an attempt to find a common ground amongst some of the biological, psychological and sociological phenomena of the obesity overeating syndromes; in Oscar Hill (Ed.) *Modern Trends in Psychosomatic Medicine*, pp.404-29, (Butterworths, London 1976).
14. Beumont, P.J.V., George, G.C.W., and Smart, D.E.: 'Dieters' and 'Vomiters' and 'Purgers' in anorexia nervosa. *Psychological Medicine* 6: 617-22 (1976).
15. Halmi, K.A., Faulk, J.P., and Schwartz, E.: Binge eating and vomiting: a survey of a college population. *Psychological Medicine*, 11: 697-706 (1981).
16. Lacey, J.H.: The patients attitude to food; in Lesoff (Ed.) *Clinical Reactions to Food*, pp.35-58 (John Wiley & Sons Ltd 1983).
17. Lacey, J.H.: The bulimic syndrome at normal body weight: Reflections on pathogenesis and clinical features. *International Journal of Eating Disorders* 2(1): 59-65 (1983).
18. Herman, P.C., and Polivy, J.: Anxiety, restraint and eating behaviour. *Journal of Abnormal Psychology* 84(6): 666-72 (1975).
19. Wardle, J., and Beinart, H.: Binge eating: A theoretical review. *British Journal of Medical Psychology* 20: 97-109 (1981).
20. Bruch, H.: *Eating Disorders, Anorexia Nervosa and the Person Within*, (Routledge and Kegan Paul, London 1974).
21. Fábry, P.: *Feeding Patterns and Nutritional Adaptions*. (Butterworths, London 1969).

22. Nisbett, R.E.: Hunger, obesity and the ventromedial hypothalamus. *Psychological Review* 79(6): 433-53 (1972).

23. Stunkard, A.J.: Biological and psychological factors in obesity; in Goodstein (Ed.) *Eating and Weight Disorders. Advances in Treatment and Research,* pp. 1-31 (Springer Publishing Co., New York 1983).

24. Wilson, G.T.: Behaviour modification and the treatment of obesity; in Stunkard (Ed.) *Obesity.* pp. 325-44 (W.B. Saunders & Co., Philadelphia 1980).

25. Slade, P.: Towards a functional analysis of anorexia nervosa and bulimia nervosa. *British Journal of Clinical Psychology* 21: 167-79 (1982).

26. Spencer, J.A., and Fremouw, W.J.: Binge eating as a function of restraint and weight classification. *Journal of Abnormal Psychology* 88(3): 262-7 (1979).

27. Pearce, J.W., Le Bow, M.D., and Orchard, J.: *The role of spouse involvement in the behavioural treatment of obese women.* Presented at the Canadian Psychological Association, Quebec City, Quebec, June 15, 1979.

28. Brownell, K.D.: Obesity: Behavioural treatments for a serious prevalent and refractory problem; in Goodstein (Ed.) *Eating and weight disorders. Advances in Treatment and Research,* pp. 71-90 (Springer Publishing Co., New York 1983).

29. Haynes, R.B., Taylor, D.W., and Sackett, D.L.: *Compliance in Health Care.* (Johns Hopkins University Press, Baltimore and London 1979).

30. Stunkard, A., Burt, V.: Obesity and the body image. II. Age at onset of disturbances in the body image. *American Journal of Psychiatry* 123(11): 1443-7 (1967).

31. Kalucy, R.S., Solow, C., Hartman, M., Crisp, A.H., McGuiness, B., and Kalucy, E.C.: Self reports of estimated body width in female obese subjects with major fat loss following ileo-jejunal bypass surgery; in Howard (Ed.) *Recent Advances in Obesity Research. 1. Proceedings of the 1st International Congress on Obesity,* pp. 331 (Newman Publishing Ltd., UK 1974).

32. Stunkard, A.J.: Psychoanalysis and Psychotherapy in *Obesity* (W.B. Saunders Company, Philadelphia 1980).

Chapter XIII

Psychiatric Aspects of Bariatric Surgery For the Control of Morbid Obesity

Obesity can be defined as the excessive accumulation of fat in various sites in the body, so that the total weight of the individual is at least 20% above that individual's ideal bodyweight. The epidemiology of obesity is interesting. In the past, obesity was generally restricted to the privileged classes and to various special individuals in society, such as chiefs. With the gradual increase in the affluence of western society, obesity has become much more of a problem, so that it has been estimated that some 1 in 3 of the population of the United States can be classified as obese.[1] Interestingly, of this large population of obese people, it has been estimated that in excess of 600 000 individuals are probably morbidly obese, morbid obesity being generally defined as a bodyweight which is more than twice the ideal weight of the individual adjusted for height, age and sex, or which exceeds that ideal weight by 50 kilograms.[2,3]

Morbid obesity presents a major health hazard.[4] Morbidly obese patients are at increased risk of developing significant physical problems, such as hypertension, coronary artery disease, and diabetes mellitis. As well, morbid obesity can exacerbate less serious physical problems.[5] Morbidly obese patients tend to have a reduced life span.[6,7] Drenick et al. in their study, assessed a group of morbidly obese males and found 11 times the mortality in the 25 to 34 year old age group, compared to a control group of average weight.[5] In the 35 to 44 year age group the study found 5 times the mortality when compared to the controls, and in the 45 to 54 year group some 3 times the mortality.

Conservative treatment of morbidly obese patients through the use of continuous diet regimens, and/or appetite suppressant tablets, can produce serious side effects. Besides, any weight loss achieved is usually impossible to maintain in the long term.[8]

Because of the failure of conservative treatment, surgical methods for controlling morbid obesity were developed. These operations have now been undertaken for the past 15 to 20 years.[9,10] The initial operations involved bypassing a large segment of bowel, the so-called jejuno-ileal bypass, and were generally associated with a significant number of complications, and a significant mortality.[11,12] Whilst these results had to be compared with the morbidity and mortality associated with morbid obesity, they were still felt to be unacceptable.

In 1980, a survey published in the United States described the outcome of jejuno-ileal or gastric bypass for morbid obesity performed on 3146 patients.[13] This survey found an 85% success rate, success being assessed as a 25% to 50% loss of the individual's excess weight. It also found a 20% to 22% morbidity, and a 2% to 3% mortality. This study certainly confirms the risks associated with the earlier operations. Whilst the study looked at all types of morbidity, it did not single out psychiatric morbidity. A psychiatric assessment of 24 patients who had undergone gastric bypass surgery 4 to 12 years previously, found that most of the complaints, both psychiatric and physical, occurred within the first 3 years after operation.[14] However, 20 patients had a good overall response, and 4 had a poor response. They found that physical and psychiatric complications were closely related. Response was assessed by them, in both physical and psychological ways, and a global rating scale was developed for this purpose.

The study undertaken by Castelnuovo-Tedesco and his group[14] found that after 3 years most patients welcomed the massive weight loss, and that psychiatric problems were associated with the development of physical problems, secondary to surgery. The study also found that most patients had gained psychologically, in terms of self-esteem, initiative, and assertiveness. They tended to become more active socially and sexually.

Other studies[15-19] have tended to confirm Castelnuovo-Tedesco's findings. However, all deal with the control of morbid obesity by gastric jejuno-ileal bypass procedures. Because of the significant morbidity of these procedures and mortality, a safer surgical operation has now been developed – bariatric surgery. This involves partitioning of the stomach through a variety of procedures. The rationale is that, by restricting the size of the stomach, the almost-universal hyperphagia of morbidly obese patients can be controlled by restricting the total intake of food. All such procedures depend, to some degree, on patient motivation and dietary compliance for a good result, as it is possible, by drinking excess high caloric fluids, or continually ingesting small quantities of high caloric food, to defeat the aim of this particular type of surgery.

To date, there have been few studies examining psychiatric aspects of bariatric surgery.[20] However, because of the apparent safety of this operation, compared to the earlier procedures, it would appear that increasing numbers of morbidly obese patients are presenting for the operation. Numerous authors have pointed out the high incidence of psychopathology in the group,[16,21] so that identification of such psychopathology would appear to be important in the assessment procedure. Patients with overt psychopathology should be excluded, as should those patients for whom the excess weight serves a particular neurotic purpose. Weight loss in the latter group can cause severe depression, and possible suicide, as opposed to the usual feelings of well-being associated with the weight loss.[22] Preoperative assessment should also help to facilitate the accurate management of psychopathology, which may be expected to emerge after operation in those patients for whom the surgery is seen as a life-saving measure.

As well, an assessment before operation could assist in identifying those patients who will have inadequate weight loss, because of non-compliance, so that more accurate exclusion criteria, aimed at this group, can be developed.

Van Itallie and Burton,[23] in discussing the dilemma of morbid obesity, felt that surgical intervention should only be considered when all other treatments undertaken seriously, and repeatedly, had failed; that prepubertal children and the elderly should be excluded and that surgery should not be attempted in the presence of excessive alcohol consumption, or serious physical illness. Moreover, they felt that a highly qualified and experienced multidisciplinary team should be assembled for the purpose of preoperative assessment, as well as extended follow-up.

This study accepts Van Itallie and Burton's recommendations, but extends them to include a psychiatric assessment that investigates those aspects of a morbidly obese individual's physical and emotional presentation, which could determine the success, or failure, of bariatric surgery.

Firstly, the clinical features of morbid obesity have been studied, in particular its duration and its association with psychopathology. Secondly, the patient's motivation for the surgery, and level of support within his, or her, immediate environment have been assessed. Finally the study investigates the feasibility of developing an assessment procedure to identify those personalities at risk for the postoperative development of psychopathology.

Methods

Some 128 patients consecutively referred for bariatric surgery at the Royal Prince Alfred Hospital, Sydney, Australia were assessed, provided that they complied with the selection criteria – morbid obesity having been present for a significant period of time, unsuccessful weight loss with dieting under medical supervision, an age range of 18 to 50 years and the absence of significant physical illness which would contraindicate surgery.

Patients came from both urban and rural areas of New South Wales. Most patients were presenting for bariatric surgery for the first time, although several had undergone a similar procedure elsewhere, the procedure having subsequently failed.

The initial assessment interview consisted of enquiring about biographic and demographic details, as well as questions about the individual's history of obesity and general physical history. A standard psychiatric history was obtained, and a formal mental status examination undertaken.

Motivation for surgery was assessed, as was the general level of support within the individual's close family, or circle of friends. If all criteria for inclusion were satisfied, the patient was informed of this by the surgeon, and a bariatric procedure carried out.

Postoperative follow-up was undertaken at regular intervals by the surgical team, who assessed the general physical status, and maintained a weight chart on each patient. The psychiatrist was only involved during this period if requested by the surgeon because of evidence of emotional disturbance, or other possible psychopathology.

Results

From March 1979 to October 1983, a total of 128 patients had been assessed for bariatric surgery. As can be seen from Table 1, of the 128, 15 were male and 113 were female. Their ages ranged from 18 to 60 years, with an average age for the males of 37 years, and for the females of 34.5 years.

The majority of patients were married, about 60% of the male patients, and almost 80% of the female patients. Approximately 60% of males had a history of life-long obesity, as opposed to late-onset obesity (commencing in adolescence, or early adult life). However, a smaller proportion, some 54% of the women, had a lifelong history of obesity – the remainder, some 46%, having a history of late-onset obesity. The duration of the obesity in this latter group ranged from 3 to 35 years, with a mean of 15.1 years. There was a positive family history of obesity in 94 of the 128 patients.

The group tended to be middle income as can be seen from Table 1. There was a large sub-group of housewives and a smaller, but significant, group of nursing sisters.

The typical patient presenting for this operation then was female, in her mid-thirties, married, and a housewife. She had a strong family history of obesity, and had been obese for at least 15 years, and often from infancy.

Table I. Patients assessed for gastroplasty (March 1979 to October 1983).

	Male (N = 15)	Female (N = 113)
Age (Years)	37 (24 to 52)	34.5 (18 to 60)
Marital Status		
Married	10	78
Single	4	22
Divorced	1	9
Widowed	–	4
Duration of Obesity		
Lifelong	11 (73.3%)	61 (54%)
Late onset	4 (26.7%)	52 (46%)
Range (Years)	15 to 25	13 to 35 (MEAN = 15.1)
Family History of Obesity	8 (53.3%)	89 (78.8%)
Occupation		
White collar	5	25
Blue collar	6	18
Nursing	–	16
Home duties	–	43
Miscellaneous	3	6
Retired	1	1
Unemployed	–	4

Psychiatric Assessment

As can be seen from Table 2, of the 128 patients, only 46 (35.9%) were felt to be uncomplicated, from the point of view of psychiatric assessment. A history of reactive depression was present in 14 and 11 had a history of psychiatric treatment, almost always for depression; 3 were currently under psychiatric care for depression. Of the patients 8 described marital stress, either past or current, usually related to the obesity. Another 6 described ongoing situational stresses of various types, for example, financial, or related to change of domicile. Six patients were referred because of doubts by the surgeon as to their motivation for surgery and another 4 patients were found by the psychiatrist to have doubtful motivation for the operation as well. Another 4 had doubtful support within the home. Five patients had a past history of significant events, or illnesses, which might possibly have affected their ability to tolerate the stress of the operation, for example, anorexia nervosa during adolescence, and loss of a child through cot death. Of the patients initially assessed, 22 were rejected for psychiatric reasons.

Table 2. Preoperative psychiatric assessment

Uncomplicated	46 (35.4%)
Psychopathology	
Past treatment	11
Current treatment	3
Reactive depression	14
Situational stress	6
Surgeon's Doubts	6
Doubtful Motivation	4
Doubtful Support	4
Miscellaneous	
(Chronic physical illness, compensation)	4
Rejections	22 (16.9%)
Total	128

Rejections

When looking at the group of patients who had been rejected, one can see from Table 3 that the reasons had largely to do with the presence of serious overt psychiatric illness (50%). These patients had been, or were currently being, seen by a psychiatrist. This group also included patients who were felt by the assessing psychiatrist to require ongoing psychiatric care. A further 3 patients were in situations of sufficient stress, of an ongoing type, to warrant their exclusion from consideration for the operation until the resolution of that stress. Sufficient motivation for surgery was lacking in 5 patients and 3 had no support within the home.

Table 3. Reasons for rejection

Overt Psychiatric Illness	11 (50%)
Severe Situational Stress	3 (13.6%)
Insufficient Motivation	5 (22.7%)
No Significant Motivation	3 (13.6%)
Total	22

Of the initial group of 22 rejections, 4 were reassessed at a later date and felt to be suitable for bariatric surgery, having responded to psychiatric treatment in the interim. Ultimately, then, 110 patients presented for gastroplasty.

Of the initial group of 128 patients, 88 had undergone bariatric surgery at the time of compiling this report, and a further 12 were awaiting surgery. Because of doubtful motivation 6 patients had dropped out preoperatively. Two were rejected during the waiting period because of the emergence of serious physical illness, and a further 2 were rejected by the surgeon because of insufficient weight loss which had been requested.

Postoperative Psychiatric Complications

As can be seen from Table 4, 14.8% of the 88 patients who had undergone surgery were referred subsequently for psychiatric assessment. Nine were seen within the first 12 months, a further 3 within the first 24 months, and 1 some 4 years after the operation. One person who had been seen before surgery, continued in psychotherapy for some 12 months after the operation.

Of the 13 patients (Table 5), 11 were seen because of depression, and 9 of these were patients whose depression was related directly, or indirectly, to the operation. A further 2 became depressed as a result of extraneous circumstances.

Table 4. Time of onset of postoperative psychiatric problems.

≤ 12 months	9
≤ 24 months	3
4 + years	1
Total	13

Table 5. Postoperative psychiatric problems.

Depression	10
Personality Disorder	1
Food Aversion	1
Sleep Deprivation	1
Total	13

One person was seen in psychotherapy because of hostile dependency personality problems, 2 were seen shortly after surgery, 1 because of a disturbance most probably related to sleep deprivation, and the other because of an aversion to semi-soft foods. All patients seen after operation have responded to psychiatric intervention. Even the person who was in psychotherapy made some gains of both an intrapersonal and interpersonal type, but lost very little weight and was considered to have an unsatisfactory result as far as the operation was concerned. Three patients continued under psychiatric care.

Interestingly, of the 11 patients seen after operation with problems in some way related to the operation, 6 had a history, prior to surgery, of psychiatric difficulties.

Discussion

This chapter presents the results of assessing a group of morbidly obese people, presenting for bariatric surgery at a large teaching hospital. As well, it presents the results of a prospective study of a group of those individuals who ultimately underwent such surgery. The assessment procedure involved a multidisciplinary team, conducting a series of interviews preoperatively, and follow-up of patients postoperatively by the surgeon and, where necessary, by the psychiatrist. Routine psychiatric follow-up was not undertaken because it was felt the problems could present at any time, and the frequency of contact, as well as the level of rapport, between the surgeon and the patients was sufficient to ensure prompt referral to the psychiatrist should emotional difficulties arise. Postoperative referral was further facilitated by the preoperative contact which patients had had with the same psychiatrist. It is anticipated, however, that formal postoperative psychiatric assessment of all patients will be undertaken after a significant period of time has elapsed.

This study confirms the high incidence of psychiatric problems, both past and current, in the morbidly obese group. The predominant problem is depression. However, there is a high incidence of intercurrent stress, both marital and situational. Although patients tend to be older, and in a stable home, and/or employment situations, their psychiatric presentation is sufficiently poor in 15.9%, or approximately 1 in 6, to lead to their rejection for bariatric surgery.

These findings tend to support the results of other studies. However, in this instance, patients were refused surgery, whereas other studies note the psychopathology without using it in their selection processes. This is most probably indicative of the fact that preoperative assessment has been biased in favour of the individual's physical status, and that psychological, and/or psychiatric assessment, has been seen as less important.

Because of the paucity of studies of patients who have undergone gastro-plasty, comparison with the earlier studies in which bypass procedures were undertaken is necessary. This shows qualitative, though not quantitative, similarities.

The findings of this study show that postoperative psychopathology is not necessarily related to physical complications. However, it does confirm that such psychopathology tends to develop within the first 12 months. It has not been possible to examine changes in more subtle, psychological parameters, such as self-image and body image, because it is felt that the follow-up should be extended for at least 5 years and a global rating scale, such as that used by Castelnuovo-Tedesco, [14] then applied.

The postoperative psychiatric referral rate of approximately 1 in 7 patients (14.8%), encompasses minor and unrelated (to surgery) problems. It attests to the comprehensive nature of the follow-up to date. Furthermore, there is little relationship between preoperative and postoperative psychiatric presentation – evidence of the usefulness of the psychiatric screening procedure. The majority of patients seen postoperatively have responded to standard psychiatric treatment and, to date, only one patient has required psychiatric intervention at longer than 2 years postoperatively. It would seem then that postoperative psychopathology may be a function of either preoperative psychiatric illness, or physical problems related to the operation. While the latter falls in the realm of the surgeon, the former can only be seen as confirming the importance of the psychiatrist in the assessment process. On the other hand, postoperative psychopathology may develop de novo, requiring assessment by a psychiatrist with experience in this area.

This study supports the feasibility of developing a standard assessment procedure to exclude persons at risk for the development of postoperative psychopathology. It would seem that important components of such a procedure are the patient's motivation for surgery, and level of close personal support, the existence of significant psychopathology or intercurrent stress and the incorporation of a sufficient waiting period before admission to hospital for surgery. At this time, it is not possible to link preoperative personality, or clinical factors, with compliance and eventual weight loss because of insufficient numbers of patients, though this study is to be undertaken.

Conclusions

This study provides clear evidence of the existence of significant psychopathology in a majority of individuals presenting for surgery for morbid obesity. Whilst such psychopathology does not necessarily exclude individuals from surgery, it makes the presence of a psychiatrist in the assessment procedure essential.

The surgeon, psychiatrist, and others in the assessment team, should be experienced in dealing with this group of patients, should develop clear-cut exclusion, as well as inclusion, criteria, and, most importantly, be available to provide follow-up well into the postoperative period.

Long-term psychological or psychiatric effects of this procedure have yet to be determined. However, this study shows gastric restrictive procedures to be associated with fewer significant psychiatric complications than the earlier procedures, and disproves the exclusive association between physical and psychiatric complaints.

It remains to be seen whether ultimate levels of weight loss can be linked to pre-morbid factors, such as motivation and compliance.

References

1. Van Itallie, T.B. and Kral, J.G.: The dilemma of morbid obesity, *Journal of the American Medical Association* 246 (9): 999-1003 (1981).
2. Metropolitan Life Insurance Company: *Mortality among overweight women.* Statistical Bulletin of the Metropolitan Life Insurance Company 41: 1 (1960).
3. Metropolitan Life Insurance Company: *Mortality among overweight men.* Statistical Bulletin of the Metropolitan Life Insurance Company. 41: 6 (1960).
4. Office of Health Economics: *Obesity and Disease* (H.M. Stationery Office, London, 1969).
5. Drenick, E.J., Bale, G.D. and Seltzer, F.: Excessive mortality and causes of death in morbidly obese men. *Journal of the American Medical Association* 243: 443-5 (1980).
6. Marks, H.H.: Influence of obesity on morbidity and mortality, *Bulletin of New York Academy of Medicine* 36: 296-9 (1960).
7. Woodhouse, S.P.: Obesity as a risk factor. *Medical Journal of Australia* spec. Suppl. 1: 11 (1969).
8. Ludbrook, J. and Jamieson, G.C.: Surgical treatment of morbid obesity, *Medical Journal of Australia* 2: 480-4 (1978).
9. Payne, J.H.; Dewind, L.T. and Commons, R.R.: Metabolic considerations in patients with jejunocolic shunts, *American Journal of Surgery* 106: 273-8 (1963).
10. Scott, H.W.; Dean, R.; Shull, H.J.; Abrams, H.S.; Webb, W.; Younger, R.K. and Brill, A.B.: New considerations in use of jejunoileal bypass in patients with morbid obesity, *Annals of Surgery* 177: 723-31 (1973).
11. Sherman, C.D.; May, A.G.; Nye, W. and Waterhouse, C.: Clinical and metabolic studies following bowel bypassing for obesity, *Annals of the New York Academy of Science* 131: 614-619 (1965).
12. Jewell, W.R.; Hermreck, A.S. and Hardin, C.A.: Complications of jejunoileal bypass for morbid obesity, *Archives of Surgery* 110: 1039-44 (1975).
13. Yates, B.Y.: Survey comparison of success, morbidity, mortality, fees and psychological benifits and costs of 3,146 patients receiving jejunoileal or gastric bypass, *American Journal of Clinical Nutrition* 33 (2 Suppl.): 513-22 (1980).
14. Castelnuovo-Tedesco, P.; Weinberg, J.; Buchanan, D.C. and Scott, H.W. Jr.: Long-term outcome of jejunoileal bypass surgery for super obesity: A psychiatric assessment, *American Journal of Psychiatry*, 139 (10): 1248-52 (1982).

15. Halmi, K.A.; Long, M.; Stunkard, A.J. and Mason, E.: Psychiatric diagnosis of morbidly obese gastric bypass patients. *American Journal of Psychiatry* 137 (4): 470-2 (1980).
16. Halmi, K.A.; Stunkard, A.J. and Mason, E.E.: Emotional responses to weight reduction by three methods: Gastric bypass, jejunoileal bypass, diet. *American Journal of Clinical Nutrition* 33 (2 Suppl.): 446-51 (1980).
17. Husemann, B. and Erzigkeit, H.: Psychological evaluation of extremely obese patients before and after surgical treatment, *World Journal of Surgery* 5: 833-8 (1981).
18. Leon, G.R.; Eckert, E.D.; Teed, E.; Varco, R.L. and Buchwald, H.: Body image, personality and life event changes after jejunoileal bypass surgery for massive obesity. *Minnesota Medicine* 63 (1): 31-4 (1980).
19. Saltzstein, E.C. and Gutmann, M.C.: Gastric bypass for morbid obesity: pre-operative and post-operative psychological evaluation of patients, *Archives of Surgery* 115 (1): 21-8 (1980).
20. Hutzler, J.C.; Keen, J.; Molinari, V. and Carey, L.: Super-obesity: A psychiatric profile of patients electing gastric stapling for the treatment of morbid obesity, *Journal of Clinical Psychiatry* 42 (12): 458-62 (1981).
21. Hopkinson, G. and Bland, R.C.: Depressive syndromes in grossly obese women, *Canadian Journal of Psychiatry* 27 (3): 213 (1982).
22. Buckwalter, J.A.: Nonsurgical factors important to the success of surgery for morbid obesity, *Surgery* 91 (1): 113-14 (1982).
23. Van Itallie, T.B. and Burton, B.T.: General summary, *American Journal of Clinical Nutrition* 33: 528-31 (1980).

Chapter XIV

The Effectiveness of some Psychological Treatments for Obesity

Introduction

The contribution of psychological concepts and methods to the study of obesity has developed rapidly both in terms of aetiological theories and of applications to treatment. The present review will be concerned with this latter aspect.

Specifically it will assess the current effectiveness of psychological treatments for obesity; assess the likely contribution of newer methods for increasing treatment effectiveness; and inquire into the possibility that applications of social psychology might have some role to play in dealing with obesity.

As with any other disorder not requiring urgent treatment there are conceptually 3 stages in treating obesity.[1] These are:

1. *recruitment* to the treatment programme;
2. *instigation* of weight loss;
3. *maintenance* of weight loss.

It is clearly possible that psychological variables and techniques which contribute to the effectiveness at one of these stages need not necessarily be effective at the other stages. An example of this would be the finding that 2-sided presentations of the case for losing weight have an effect on recruitment,[2] but not on the instigation or maintenance of weight loss.[3,4] A further example is that the addition of medication to the early stages of a behavioural programme leads to greater weight loss in the instigation phase, but poorer maintenance of that weight loss.[5]

On theoretical grounds it might be expected that social psychological variables would be particularly important in the recruitment and instigation phases. Hence their inclusion in this review.

Also the role of personality and mood factors in obesity will be briefly reviewed.

Current Effectiveness of Psychological and Other Treatments

The decades of the 1960s and 1970s saw an explosion of research into the effectiveness of new psychological and other treatments for obesity. The effectiveness of these new treatments has been assessed in numerous reviews[1,6-12].

These reviewers have used a number of different methods for summarizing the data reviewed, the main ones being: a) mean weight loss; and b) proportions of clients losing more than a stated number of kilograms in weight.

Table 1 summarizes the results of these reviews in terms of crude unweighted means of mean weight losses reported in the literature for major categories of treatment procedures. These means are reported to the nearest 0.5 kilogram. The data used on behavioural procedures, minimal treatment plus diet, and commercial weight loss groups are derived from Ley,[1] data on hypnosis from Wadden and Anderton,[10] and on exercise from Epstein and Wing[7] and Thompson et al.[9]

Needless to say several caveats are in order in interpreting the table. Lengths of treatment and follow-up have varied considerably, degree of overweight in those treated has ranged from mild to massive obesity; within samples, distributions of weight loss have often been heavily skewed; finally, within treatments, mean weight losses have often varied considerably. For example in the investigations of Ley and his associates,[3,13] and Skilbeck et al.,[4] mean weight losses in large groups of clients recruited in the same way but in 2 different years, and exposed to the same treatment were 3.36kg and 5.58kg at 8-week follow-up.

Table 1. Mean weight losses for different methods of treating obesity.

		Attention/drug placebo	2.7
Exercise	1.4	Psychotherapy	4.5
Hypnosis	2.3	Miminal treatment plus diet	5.0
Aversion therapy	2.7	Behavioural self control	5.9
Contingency management	2.7	Commercial weight loss group	8.6

Table 2. Weight losses achieved by various treatments for obesity.

Method	Percentage of studies showing mean weight loss of 4.5kg or more (N. of studies in parentheses)	Proportion of clients losing 9kg or more	
		Wing and Jeffery[6]	Ley
Aversive conditioning	33% (9)	–	–
Contingency management	21% (14)	–	–
Self-control procedures	73% (26)	–	33%
Behaviour modification	–	16%	–
Commercial groups	100% (7)	–	34%
Psychoanalysis	–	–	28%
Hypnosis	11% (9)	–	–
Exercise	3% (29)	–	–
Anorectic drugs	–	19%	–
Hormones	–	24%	–
Medication	56% (25)	–	36%
Diet	–	25%	27%

To partially overcome these problems Ley reported data on the number of investigations of a given treatment reporting mean weight losses of 4.5kg or more and 4kg or less, and the percentage of clients losing over 4.5kg, 9kg or 13.6kg,[1] while Wing and Jeffery reported the percentage of clients losing 9kg or more.[6] These data together with those on exercise from Epstein and Wing,[7] and on hypnosis from Wadden and Anderton,[10] are shown in Table 2.

The results confirm those shown in Table 1 in rank ordering techniques. Hypnosis, exercise, aversion therapy, and contingency management seem very ineffective while self-control, diet and drugs seem to be effective treatments as does attendance at commercial weight loss groups. Thus at least some treatments are useful in the instigation of weight loss. This raises the obvious question of the maintenance of these effects. Ley [1] concluded that for diet, self-control and semi-starvation procedures, about 20% of clients would lose 9kg or more and keep it off for more than 12 months. Foreyt *et al.* reviewed all studies of behavioural procedures which provided data on follow-up at 12 months or more and found that mean weight loss at the end of treatment was 6kg and at 12-month follow-up mean loss was also 6kg. [8] In 12 of the 16 studies reviewed mean weight loss at follow-up was 4.5kg or more.

The position at the end of the 1970s was, then, that there were available a number of procedures which had a high probability of producing a mean weight loss of 4.5kg or more and of maintaining that weight loss for 12 months or more. Even the more stringent criterion of losing 9kg or more would be achieved by some 30% of clients and about 20% of clients would maintain their 9kg loss for a year or more. Whether weight losses of this magnitude would be clinically or even cosmetically significant would of course depend on the individual case, but it was obvious that the technology did not seem capable of ensuring that most obese clients would achieve their ideal weights.

Schachter's data

Because the success rates for treatments, although real, were limited there was some pessimism abroad about the likelihood of being able to help the overweight to slim. This pessimism was reinforced by the increasing evidence of the role of biological factors in obesity.[14-17]

However, Schachter[18] presented data which cast some doubt on the validity of the pessimistic view. Schachter reported on a relatively informal survey of 2 samples of people. One consisted of 83 members of the Psychology Department at Columbia Univeristy (faculty, secretaries, technicians, and graduate students), and the other of 78 persons working in Amagansett, Long Island, New York, where Schachter was wont to spend his vacations.

Of the 46 people in the sample who had at some time or other been obese (15% or more overweight) 40 had tried to lose weight. Approximately 72% had successfully reduced themselves to normal or near-normal weight without professional help. The average weight losses for all of those who tried were 12kg for males and 11kg for females. Those who managed to bring themselves down to normal weight lost 13kg (females) and 17.7kg (males).

Thus the majority of those who had tried to lose weight had been successful. Further, mean weight losses achieved were substantial in relation to those reported in the literature.

Schachter had of course pointed out the dangers of generalizing too much from a sample of this nature, but if the findings can be confirmed by studies of more adequate samples, then it would seem that professionals are probably dealing with a rather atypical group of obese persons, i.e. those whose own efforts at weight loss have been unsuccessful.

Attempts to increase the effectiveness of available treatments

Recent attempts to increase the effectiveness of treatments have included:
  1. the use of large financial incentives in contingency contracts;
  2. the involvement of others who are significant to the client;
  3. the combination of treatments.

The first of these is well exemplified in the work of Jeffery et al.,[19,20] and Wing et al.[21]

Jeffery et al.[19] collected $200 deposits whose return was contingent on weight loss and obtained a mean weight loss of 9kg in the group so treated. Wing et al.[19] made their clients deposit $225. In 2 different groups studied mean weight losses of 10.4kg and 8.5kg were obtained at 3-month follow-up. In a subsequent study the deposit requested from clients by Jeffery et al. was $300.[20] Mean weight loss achieved at the end of treatment was 14.5kg dropping to 6.4kg at the end of 12-month follow-up.

These results look quite promising, but the technique has an unfortunate drawback. In the sample studied by Jeffery et al. only 43% of those offered treatment in the $300 deposit condition agreed to participate.

The involvement of significant others has in the case of children included a parent or both parents as targets for weight loss techniques as well as their obese child. Research by Kingsley and Shapiro,[22] and Epstein et al.,[7,23] suggests that this technique is not effective, in that these investigations found no greater weight loss than when the child alone was the target.

With adults attempts have been made to involve the spouse in the treatment programme. Brownell et al. reported a highly significant effect for this technique.[24] At the end of 10 weeks a spouse-involvement group had lost 9kg as opposed to the 5.5kg lost by a group without spouse involvement. These differences were maintained at 12-month follow-up, when mean weight loss in the spouse-involvement group was found to be 13.6kg and in the treated-alone group 9kg. Further, 67% of the spouse-involvement group lost 9kg or more as opposed to only 44% of the group treated alone.

Unfortunately, this spectacular success has not been confirmed in other studies. Wilson and Brownell found only an insignificant difference for spouse involvement (4.5kg opposed to 3.6kg weight loss) at the end of 8 weeks treatment, with the treated-alone group actually losing more weight by 6-month follow-up (6kg as opposed to 3.2kg).[25]

This failure to find an effect for spouse involvement was echoed in the investigation of Brownell and Stunkard who found weight loss in a spouse-involved group to be 9kg after 6 months treatment dropping to 4.5kg at 12-month follow-up, as opposed to losses of 7.7kg and 4kg at these times by a treated-alone group.[26] Finally, Murphy et al. obtained mean weight losses at end of treatment of 7.6kg and 8.2kg[27] in spouse-involved clients as compared with 7kg and 7.2kg for treated-alone clients. However, at follow-up the spouse-involvement clients showed mean losses of 8.6kg and 5.4kg at 1 year, and 7.3kg and 3.2kg at 2 years. Corresponding figures for those treated-alone clients were at 1 year 3.6kg and 3.2kg, and at 2 years a gain of 2.7kg and a loss of 2.7kg.

Combinations of treatments have involved either behaviour modification and a very restricted kilojoule intake, or behaviour modification and medication.

Lindner and Blackburne[28] and Musante[29] both reported impressive results for the first of these combinations. Of the clients, 34% lost more than 18kg and another 33% lost 9kg or more. Thus altogether two-thirds lost over 9kg. These studies, however, suffered from a lack of detail about follow-up results.

More recently Miller and Sims have reported on a similar low-kilojoule (3000) plus behaviour modification regimen.[30] This programme is similar to the previously mentioned ones and included a 12-month follow-up. At 12 months mean weight loss was 13.2kg and 66% of subjects had lost 9kg or more.

Combinations of medication and behavioural techniques were investigated by Craighead et al.[5] Medication alone had, by the end of the 6-month treatment period, resulted in a mean weight loss of 6kg and behaviour therapy alone to a mean loss of 11kg. The 2 treatments combined resulted in a mean weight loss of 15.4kg. Another combination – Rogerian group psychotherapy and medication – resulted in a mean weight loss of 14.5kg. However at 1-year follow-up behaviour therapy alone (9kg) proved superior to behaviour therapy plus medication (4.5kg) and to Rogerian therapy plus medication (6.4kg). Thus the short-term improvement achieved by the addition of medication seemed to be at the expense of a greater relapse when treatment finished.

Brownell and Stunkard also reported high weight loss in a group treated by a combination of fenfluramine and behaviour therapy.[26] This group lost an average of 10kg.

Other Possible Contributions from Psychology

Attempts to improve on the current effectiveness of behavioural and psychological treatments could in theory utilize findings from a) the study of individual differences, and b) the social psychological findings concerning persuasive communications. These would be in addition to such commonsense approaches as making treatment easier for the obese by providing it at the workplace,[31] or school,[32] or even by correspondence course.[33] These 3 strategies would not be expected to produce greater weight loss, but, by making treatment more accessible or less costly, would be expected to reduce drop-out and/or widen the pool of potential participants.

In contrast the systematic use of individual differences and persuasive communication variables might lead to increased weight loss. Evidence on these topics will now be considered.

Individual differences and weight loss

Because historically[34] obesity has often been regarded as the result of personality difficulties, there has been research into the personality characteristics of the

obese. The initial expectations were that the obese would be more anxious and/
or more depressed than their leaner peers. If this were found to be so, then
treatment effectiveness could presumably be increased by dealing with the problems of anxiety and depression experienced by the obese. Most research has been
conducted with small samples of obese subjects attending clinics or receiving
hospital treatment for their condition. There are usually no adequate controls
and there are other methodological faults.[1] Better quality investigations using
community samples have found lower depression,[35,36] no differences in
neuroticism[35] and lower anxiety in the obese.[36] However Ley reported a positive
correlation between degree of overweight and measures of both anxiety and
depression.[13,38]

The findings of no increases in depression led some theorists to propose that
the obese were less depressed because obesity was a successful defence against
depression. If this is so then the expectation would be that to lose weight would
be to lose the defence and thus depression would emerge. Stunkard and Rush
reviewed the literature and found a great deal of anecdotal and clinical evidence
to support this notion.[39] However, the studies reviewed were methodologically
unsound, and failed to control for: a) effects of restricted kilojoule intake per se;
b) effects of hospitalization; c) self-selection of subjects.

Investigations into the relationship between changes in weight and depression have not found evidence to support the hypothesis that obesity is a defence
against depression. A small study by Taylor *et al.* found no increase in depression
in 22 subjects at the Stanford Eating Disorders Clinic.[40] Wing *et al.*, in an investigation of 76 clients, found that decreases in weight were accompanied by
significant decreases in depression and anxiety.[41] Another large investigation[38]
found that: a) there were correlations between degree of overweight and depression; b) weight loss was accompanied by a drop in depression; c) the greater the
weight loss the greater the drop in depression. This investigation involving 327
obese females therefore yielded strong evidence against the hypothesis that obesity is a defence against depression.

Further, neither anxiety nor depression as measured by the Multiple Affect
Adjective Checklist, nor extraversion nor neuroticism is a good predictor of
eventual weight loss.[13] Wing *et al.* also report no relation between initial mood
and subsequent weight loss.[41] However, in 2 large-scale series the personal control subscale of the Rotter Internal-External Control Measure has been found to
be correlated with weight loss.[42,43] These results are summarized in Table 3.

The other main variable associated with weight loss is gender. Men lose
weight more easily than women.[1] Interestingly enough men's weights vary more
cross-culturally than women's weights. Thus, while there was no significant difference between the proportion of women judged obese in cultures which value
slimness and those that value fatness in women, obesity rates for men varied
significantly cross-culturally[16] A possible interpretation of this finding is that

Table 3. Correlations between weight loss, mood and personality.

Investigation	Sample size	Correlation with weight loss at stated follow-up			
		2 weeks	4 weeks	8 weeks	16 weeks
1. Ley[13]	136				
a) MAACL Depression		−0.10	−0.01	+0.03	+0.04
b) MAACL Anxiety		−0.04	−0.05	−0.04	+0.09
2. Ley et al.[3]	131				
a) MPI Neuroticism		–	–	−0.08	–
b) MPI Extraversion		–	–	+0.06	–
3. Ley[13]	136				
a) MPI Neuroticism		–	–	−0.25*	–
b) MPI Extraversion		–	–	+0.09	–
4. Kincey[42]	131				
Internal control		+0.03	+0.12	+0.31*	–
5. Kincey[43]	136				
Internal control		–	–	+ 0.24*	–

(* p < 0.05)

obesity rates in men are more responsive to environmental factors, which makes it easier for them to lose weight.

However, it is clear that the study of personality and mood variables is, in its present state, unable to offer advice in methods of increasing or maintaining weight loss.

Social psychology and treatment effectiveness

The use of fear appeals to motivate compliance with recommended health practices has been fairly common. Sutton reviewed 38 such investigations and concluded that fear appeals have an effect on both intentions and behaviour.[44] The only studies on obesity reviewed were those of Ley and his collaborators.[3,4,13] These investigators found that the effects of fear appeals on weight loss depended upon: a) degree of fear aroused; b) the position of the fear appeal in relation to recommendations about diet; and c) whether there was a single or a multiple exposure to the fear message. Weight loss had a curvilinear relationship to degree of fear aroused. Subjects who were moderately frightened by the message lost more weight than those who were little or highly frightened. The fear appeal was most effective when placed just before recommendations for action. Finally a single exposure to the frightening message was more effective than multiple exposures. These results are summarized in Table 4.

Table 4. Effects of manipulation of fear appeals on weight loss.

Investigation		Mean weight loss (kg) at	
		8 weeks	16 weeks
1. *Judged degree of likely fear arousal*			
Ley et al. [3]	Low	3.1	–
	Medium	3.7 (ns)	–
	High	3.5	–
Skilbeck et al.[4]	Low	6.7	7.44
	Medium	4.9 (ns)	7.39
	High	6.3	8
2. *Degree of fear aroused*			
Skilbeck et al.[4]	Low	5.4	6.5
	Medium	7.1 (p < 0.01)	9.3 (p < 0.05)
	High	4.8	6.6
3. *Exposure to fear appeal*			
Skilbeck et al.[4]	Single	6.6	8.8
	Multiple	5.3 (ns)	6.3 (p < 0.01)
4. *Position of fear appeal*			
Skilbeck et al.[4]	a) before, but separated from, recommendation:		
		4	5.5
	b) Immediately before recommendation:		
		5.9 (p < 0.05)	8.5 (ns)
	c) After recommendation:		
		4.7	8.1

Table 5. Probability of drop-out at a given follow-up in relation to weight loss achieved at the previous follow-up session.

Weight loss previous session	Cut off in kg for			Probability of drop-out		
	2 weeks	4 weeks	8 weeks	4 weeks	8 weeks	16 weeks
Quartile						
First	1.4 or less	1.8 or less	3.2 or less	0.11	0.32	0.49
Second	1.8-2.3	2.3-2.7	3.6-4.5	0.16	0.32	0.40
Third	2.7-3.2	3.2-4.1	5-5.9	0.09	0.19	0.36
Fourth	3.6-5.9	4.5-7.3	6.4-10.9	0.04	0.12	0.18

From these results it would appear that presenting fear appeals in the correct way leads to mean differences in weight loss of between 1.8kg and 3.2kg between best and worst conditions. As it can be argued that continued compliance with a weight reduction programme is reinforced by weight loss, mean differences of this order can in theory be valuable.

Data suggesting that weight loss reinforces continuance in weight reduction programmes is presented in Table 5, which is based on the investigations reviewed by Ley.[13] Over 300 clients were involved.

It can be seen that probability of attendance at a session is quite well predicted by relative success is losing weight up to the time of the previous session. In fact, obese women whose weight loss was below the median had double the drop-out rate of those whose weight loss was above median. While other interpretations of these data are possible, they are consistent with the hypothesis that success in losing weight reinforces compliance with weight loss programmes.

Other social psychological variables which have been investigated included sidedness of communication. Two-sided communications have not proved successful in increasing weight loss,[3,13] but have been shown to affect probability of volunteering to participate in a slimming programme.[2] Of the overweight members of a general practice sample who received a two-sided message, 87% expressed an interest in joining a scheme as compared with 68% of those who received a one-sided message.

Correlational data have also been reported which support the Fishbein and Ajzen model of attitude and behaviour change.[13,45] To date no interventions have been attempted using this model but there are obvious possibilities for devising such interventions. Similarly, correlational data supportive of the Health Belief Model have been reported.[46,47] Once more there is a lack of research into attempts to use the model to improve treatment effectiveness.

At this stage it would appear that social psychological models and findings might have some application in increasing the effectiveness of treatments for obesity. Research will show whether this promised potential can be realized.

Conclusions

It looks as though it is not difficult to obtain mean weight losses of 5.5kg or so and maintain them for a year.

Some combined treatments, especially those involving medication, show a greater initial weight loss – 9kg to 13.6kg – but the effects seem to be short lived and at the end of a year mean weight loss seems to be about 5.5kg.

The greatest weight losses which are sustained seem to result from semi-residential programmes combining strict control of food intake with behavioural procedures, of some weeks' duration where intake is reduced to well below 4000 kilojoules. With these regimens about two-thirds of patients lose and keep off more than 9kg. This compares very favourably with the 20% keeping off 9kg for a year or more obtained by other psychological methods.

The dangers in drawing too strong a conclusion are of course the usual ones. There are still too few investigations available, and there is the likelihood that the more stringent a treatment package is, the more likely it is that more people will refuse it. It possibly becomes, in effect, a selection device for picking the most highly motivated people.

Schachter's result is also worth remembering. Many, if not most, people can succeed in losing weight without professional help and their reported weight loss of 9kg or more on average is obviously a very good result.

But clearly if we have to choose which is the most successful non-invasive current technique it must be a combination of a period of severe kilojoule restriction combined with behavioural procedures.

With the growing emphasis on the probable role of biological factors in the genesis, maintenance and relapse rates in obesity[1,14-17] it can be expected that over the next decade treatments will be evolved which take more account of these factors.

Even without these developments however it would be unwise to be too despondent about the chances of successfully losing weight. If Schachter is right, about two-thirds will be successful by their own efforts, and the rest can, with professional help, expect a mean weight loss of 6kg or so, with about a third losing 9kg or more.

Finally, it is possible that the application of social psychological findings will make some impact on weight reduction, at least in the short term during the recruitment and instigation phases.

References

1. Ley, P.: The psychology of obesity; Rachman (Ed) Contributions to Medical Psychology 2. (Pergamon Press, Oxford, 1980).
2. Ley, P., Whitworth, M.A., Woodward, R., and Yorke, R.: Effects of sidedness and fear arousal on willingness to volunteer for a slimming programme. Health Education Journal 36: 67-9 (1977).
3. Ley, P., Bradshaw, P.W., Kincey, J.A., Couper-Smartt, H.J., and Wilson, M.: Psychological variables in the control of obesity; Burland, Samuel, and Yudkin (Eds) Obesity (Churchill-Livingstone, London 1974).
4. Skilbeck, C.E., Tulips, J.G., and Ley, P.: Effects of fear arousal, fear exposure and sidedness on compliance with dietary instruction. European Journal of Social Psychology 7: 221-49 (1977).
5. Craighead, L.W., Stunkard, A.J. and O'Brien, R.: Behaviour therapy and pharmacotherapy of obesity. Lancet 2: 1045-7 (1980).
6. Wing, R., and Jeffery, R.W.: Out-patient treatment of obesity: a comparison of methodology and clinical results. International Journal of Obesity 3: 261-79 (1979).
7. Epstein, L.H., and Wing, R.R.: Aerobic exercise and weight. Addictive Behaviors 5: 371-88 (1980).

8. Foreyt, J.P., Goodrick, G.D. and Gotto, A.M.: Limitations of behavioral treatments of obesity: Review and analysis. *Journal of Behavioral Medicine* 4: 159-74 (1981).

9. Thompson, J.K., Jarvie, G.H., Lahey, B.B. and Cureton, K.J.: Exercise and obesity: etiology, physiology and intervention. *Psychological Bulletin* 91: 55-79 (1982).

10. Wadden, T.A., and Anderton, C.H.: The clinical use of hypnosis. *Psychological Bulletin,* 91: 215-43 (1982).

11. Brownell, K.D.: Obesity: Understanding a serious, prevalent and refractory problem. *Journal of Consultiny and Clinical Psychology* 50: 820-40 (1982).

12. Brownell, K.D. The addictive disorders. In Franks, Wilson, Kendall and Brownell (Eds) *Annual Review of Behaviour Therapy.* Vol. 8. (Guilford Press, New York 1982).

13. Ley, P.: Psychological and behavioural factors in weight loss. In Bray (Ed.) *Recent Advances in Obesity Research. II.* (Newman, London 1978).

14. Wooley, S.C., Wooley, O.W. and Dyrenforth, S.R.: Theoretical, practical and social issues in the behavioral treatment of obesity. *Journal of Applied Behavior Analysis* 12: 3-25 (1979).

15. Stunkard, A.J.: Biological and psychological factors in obesity; in Goodstein (Ed.) *Eating and weight disorders* (Springer, New York 1982).

16. Ley, P.: Psychological, social and cultural determinants of acceptable fatness; in Turner (Ed) *Nutrition and lifestyles.* (Applied Science Press, London 1980).

17. Storlien, L.H.: Animal models of obesity. In Bond (Ed.) *Animal Models of Psychopathology* (Academic Press, Sydney 1984).

18. Schachter, S.: Recidivism and self cure of smoking and obesity. *American Psychologist* 37: 436-44 (1982).

19. Jeffery, R.W., Thompson, P.D. and Wing, R.R.: Effects on weight reduction of strong monetary contracts. *Behavior Research and Therapy* 16: 363-9 (1978).

20. Jeffery, R.W., Gerber, W.M., Rosenthal, B.S. and Lindquist, R.A.: Monetary contracts in weight control : effectiveness of group and individual contracts of varying sizes. *Journal of Consulting and Clinical Psychology* 51: 242-8 (1983).

21. Wing, R.R., Epstein, L.H., Marcus, M. and Shapira, B.: Strong monetary contingencies for weight loss during treatment and maintenance. *Behavior Therapy* 12: 702-10 (1981).

22. Kingsley, R.W. and Shapiro, J.A.: A comparison of three behavioural programs for the control of obesity in children. *Behavioural Therapy* 8: 30-6 (1977).

23. Epstein, L.H., Wing, R.R., Koeske, R., Andrasik, F. and Ossip, D.J.: Child and parent weight loss in family based behaviour modification programs. *Journal of Consulting and Clinical Psychology* 49: 674-85 (1981).

24. Brownell, K.D., Heckerman, C.L., Westlake, R.J., Hayes, S.C. and Monti, P.M.: The effect of couples training and partner cooperativeness in the behavioural treatment of obesity. *Behavior Research and Therapy* 16: 323-33 (1978).

25. Wilson, G.T. and Brownell, K.D.: Behaviour therapy for obesity; Including family members in the treatment process. *Behavior Therapy* 9: 943-5 (1978).

26. Brownell, K.D. and Stunkard, A.J.: Couples training, pharmacotherapy and behavior therapy in the treatment of obesity. *Archives of General Psychiatry* 38: 1224-9 (1981).

27. Murphy, J.K., Williamson, D.A., Buxton, A.E., Moody, N.A. and Warner, M.: Long term effects of spouse involvement on weight loss and maintenance. *Behavior Therapy* 13: 681-93 (1982).

28. Lindner, P.G. and Blackburn, G.L.: Multi-disciplinary approach to obesity, utilizing fasting modified by protein sparing therapy. *Obesity and bariatric Medicine* 5: 198-216 (1976).

29. Musante, G.J.: The dietary rehabilitation Clinic: evaluation report of a behavioral and dietetic treatment of obesity. *Behavior Therapy* 7: 198-204 (1976).

30. Miller, P.M. and Sims, K.L.: Evaluation and component analysis of a comprehensive weight control program. *International Journal of Obesity* 5: 57-65 (1981).

31. Abrams, D.B. and Follick, M.J.: (1983). Behavioral weight loss intervention at the worksite. *Journal of Consulting and Clinical Psychology* 51: 226-33 (1983).

32. Lansky, D. and Vance, M.A.: School based intervention for adolescent obesity. *Journal of Consulting and Clinical Psychology,* 51: 147-8 (1983).

33. Jeffery, R.W. and Gerber, W.M.: Group and correspondence treatment for weight reduction. *Behavior Therapy* 13: 24-30 (1982).

34. Bruch, H.: *Eating disorders.* Basic Books, New York (1973).

35. Simon, R.I.: Obesity as a depressive equivalent. *Journal of the American Medical Association* 183: 134-6 (1963).

36. Crisp, A.H. and McGuiness, B.: Jolly fat: relation between obesity and psychoneurosis in the general population. *British Medical Journal* 1: 7-10 (1976).

37. Silverstone, J.T.: Psychosocial aspects of obesity. *Proceedings of the Royal Society of Medicine* 61: 371-2 (1968).

38. Ley, P.: Some tests of the hypothesis that obesity is a defence against depression. *Behavior Research and Therapy* 22: 197-9 (1984).

39. Stunkard, A.J. and Rush, J.: Dieting and depression re-examined. *Annals of Internal Medicine* 81: 526-33 (1974).

40. Taylor, C.B., Ferguson, J.M. and Reading, J.C.: Gradual weight loss and depression. *Behavior Therapy* 9: 622-5 (1978).

41. Wing, R.R., Marcus, M.D., Epstein, L.H. and Kupfer, D.: Mood and weight loss in a behavioural treatment program. *Journal of Consulting and Clinical Psychology* 51: 153-5 (1983).

42. Kincey, J.A.: Internal-external control and weight loss in the obese. *Journal of Clinical Psychology* 37: 100-3 (1981).

43. Kincey, J.A.: *Internal-external control, obesity and health education.* Health Education Council (London) Occasional Paper (1984).

44. Sutton, S.R.: Fear arousing communications: a critical examination of research and theory. In Eiser (Ed.) *Social Psychology and Behavioural Medicine* (Wiley, New York 1982).

45. Sejwacz, D., Ajzen, I. and Fishbein, M.: Predicting and understanding weight loss; in Ajzen and Fishbein (Eds) *Understanding attitudes and predicting social behavior.* (Prentice Hall, Englewood Cliffs 1980).

46. Becker, M.H.: Understanding patient compliance; in Cohen (Ed.) *New directions in patient compliance.* (Lexington Books, Lexington 1979).

47. Becker, M.H., Maiman, L.A., Kirscht, J.P., Haefner, D.P., Drachman, R.H., and Taylor, D.W.: Patient perceptions and compliance: recent studies of the Health Belief Model; in Haynes, Taylor, Sackett (Eds) *Compliance in health care.* (Johns Hopkins University Press, Baltimore 1979).

Appendix A

EVA (eating visual analogue) Questionnaire

Example:

Do you like eating food?

never .... always

If you like eating food most of the time you will put a mark on the line between the mid-point and always. The more often you like eating food the closer to always you will put the line.

Do you think about food?

Item
1   never 0 .... 10 always

Do you weigh the food you eat?

2   always 10 ....0 never

Do you count calories?

3   never 0 .... 10 always

Do you read recipes?

4   always 10 ....0 never

Do you feel you have control
over how much you eat?

5   never 10 .... 0 always

Do you always eat everything
that is on your plate?

6   always 0 ....10 never

Do you weigh yourself?

7   always 10 ....0 never

Do you find thoughts of food
going round in your mind?

8   never 0 .... 10 always

Do you collect recipes?

9   never 0 .... 10 always

Do you talk a lot about food

10   never 0 .... 10 always

Do you diet?

11   always 10 ....0 never

Do you try to control
your weight?

12   never 0 .... 10 always

Do you go on eating
binges?

13   always 10 ....0 never

Do you feel that you are
overweight?

14   always 10 ....0 never

If you look at yourself in a mirror,
would you think that you look overweight?

15   always 10 ....0 never

Do you wish to change the shape of
parts of your body?

16   always 10 ....0 never

Do you feel hungry?

17   never 0 .... 10 always

Do you feel that your body build is a
disadvantage to you?

18   never 0 .... 10 always

Do you find it very difficult to control
your body weight?

19   never 0 .... 10 always

Index